Microvascular Tissue Transfer in the Head and Neck Region

Friedrich Bootz and Gottfried H. Müller

with the collaboration of
Michael Ehrenfeld

Foreword by P. M. Stell

192 illustrations, most in color

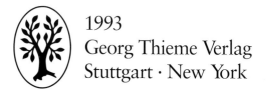

1993
Georg Thieme Verlag
Stuttgart · New York

Thieme Medical Publishers, Inc.
New York

Priv.-Doz. Dr. F. Bootz
Leitender Oberarzt der
Universitäts-Hals-Nasen-Ohren-Klinik
(ENT Department)
Silcherstraße 5
D-72076 Tübingen

Prof. Dr. G. H. Müller
Chefarzt der Chirurgischen Klinik
(Dept. of Surgery)
Caritas-Krankenhaus
Wachbacher Straße 52
D-97980 Bad Mergentheim

Priv.-Doz. Dr. Dr. M. Ehrenfeld
Leitender Oberarzt der
Klinik und Poliklinik für Kiefer- und
Gesichtschirurgie der Universität Tübingen
(Maxillofacial Surgery Dept.)
Osianderstraße 2–8
D-72076 Tübingen

Translated by Conny Huthsteiner, M. D.

Library of Congress Cataloging-in-Publication Data

Bootz, Friedrich.
  [Mikrovaskuläre Gewebetransplantation im Kopf-Hals-Bereich.
English]
  Microvascular tissue transfer in the head and neck region /
Friedrich Bootz and Gottfried H. Müller : with the collaboration of
Michael Ehrenfeld.
      p. cm.
  Includes bibliographical references and index.
  ISBN 3-13-112101-7. – – ISBN 0-86577-503-6
  1. Head--Surgery.   2. Neck--Surgery.   3. Free flaps (Surgery).
4. Surgery, Plastic.   5. Microsurgery.   I. Müller, Gottfried H.
II. Ehrenfeld, M. (Michael) III. Title.
  [DNLM: 1. Head--surgery.   2. Neck--surgery.   3. Microsurgery-
-methods.   4. Tissue Transplantation--methods.   5. Vascular Surgery-
-methods.   6. Surgical Flaps--methods.   WE 705 8725m 1993a]
RD521.B5613   1993
617.5'1059--dc20
DNLM/DLC   93-8837
for Library of Congress   CIP

This book is an authorized translation of the German edition; published and copyrighted 1992 by Georg Thieme Verlag, Stuttgart, Germany.
Title of the German edition: Mikrovaskuläre Gewebetransplantation im Kopf-Hals-Bereich.

© 1993 Georg Thieme Verlag,
Rüdigerstraße 14, D-70469 Stuttgart, Germany
Thieme Medical Publishers, Inc.,
381 Park Avenue South, New York, N.Y. 10016

Typesetting by Setzerei Lihs

Printed in Germany by K. Grammlich GmbH

ISBN 3-13-112101-7 (GTV, Stuttgart)
ISBN 0-86577-503-6 (TMP, New York)

Important Note:
Medicine is an ever-changing science undergoing continual development. Research and clinical experience are continually expanding our knowledge, in particular our knowledge of proper treatment and drug therapy. Insofar as this book mentions any dosage or application, readers may rest assured that the authors, editors and publishers have made every effort to ensure that such references are in accordance with the state of knowledge at the time of production of the book.
Nevertheless this does not involve, imply, or express any guarantee or responsibility on the part of the publishers in respect of any dosage instructions and forms of application stated in the book. Every user is requested to examine carefully the manufacturers' leaflets accompanying each drug and to check, if necessary in consultation with a physician or specialist, whether the dosage schedules mentioned therein or the contraindications stated by the manufacturers differ from the statements made in the present book. Such examination is particularly important with drugs that are either rarely used or have been newly released on the market. Every dosage schedule or every form of application used is entirely at the user's own risk and responsibility. The authors and publishers request every user to report to the publishers any discrepancies or inaccuracies noticed.

Foreword

It is a great honor to write a word of welcome and recommendation for this book. I have read it with great interest, and I have been very impressed by its careful and thorough cover of what has now become a very important field for the head and neck oncologist. There may be debates about the relative value of individual techniques, but there can be no doubt that microvascular tissue transfer has found a permanent niche in this field of surgery. In this book both the beginner and the more experienced surgeon will find reliable guidelines to all the common and important techniques.

Dr. Bootz and Dr. Müller have approached microvascular surgery from different starting points: Dr. Bootz from that of the ENT surgeon, Dr. Müller from that of general surgery. One of the strengths of this book derives from this fruitful co-operation. It is also a particular pleasure for me to have played a small part in the training of Dr. Bootz.

York, Spring 1993   *P. M. Stell*

Preface

In the last few years, microvascular tissue transfer has become a standard procedure of reconstructive surgery. At first, this particular operative technique was used primarily by plastic surgeons in the reconstruction of certain parts of the body, but soon, mainly through intradisciplinary cooperation, it was picked up by head and neck surgeons as well.

We, the authors of this volume, come from different disciplines: ENT, general, and maxillofacial surgery. The contents and structure of this book reflect our experiences in many years of successful cooperation. It is intended to be a concrete, practical guide to microvascular tissue transfer in the head and neck area, including step-by-step descriptions of the necessary techniques to those who wish to learn them.

In the Introduction, prerequisites for microvascular surgery, including suggestions for training and practice, are discussed. The next chapter (Technique of harvesting flaps) describes the most important and most frequently used tissue transfers, for example, fasciocutaneous, myocutaneous, and osteomyocutaneous flaps. Only those flaps with which we have experience and which in our opinion satisfy all requirements of reconstruction in the head and neck area are described. We purposely chose illustrations that allowed us to describe specific operative techniques in the legends, so that the reader is not required to read long narrative passages. Thus, the book is also useful as a reference source.

The chapter on Clinical Applications includes our experiences with free tissue transfer for reconstructive purposes in the head and neck region. In order to avoid listing a confusingly large number of different flaps for various reconstructions, we placed particular emphasis on the use of a standardized procedure. We believe that it is important for a successful treatment of the patient that the surgeon master only a few flap harvesting techniques. The goal of the reconstructive surgeon should not be to learn the greatest number of different flap techniques possible since the lack of extensive experience with each one will endanger the success of each application.

At the end of the book, complications are discussed, which are usually manageable if they are detected early enough. Since, for example, complications of the vessel anastomosis cause the failure of the entire tissue transfer, it is especially important that the surgeon know ways of avoiding complications as well as dealing with postoperative problems.

The concept and contents of this book are suitable for the beginner as an introduction to microvascular tissue transfer and for the experienced surgeon as a reference source.

Tübingen and Bad Mergentheim, *F. Bootz*
Spring 1993 *G. H. Müller*

Contents

1 Introduction

In the last few years microvascular tissue transfers have become common in reconstructive surgery of the head and neck.

As early as 1959 the first free tissue transfer was carried out by Seidenberg and coworkers who used a jejunal transplant to reconstruct the hypopharynx and cervical esophagus. Free flaps were developed further in the 1970s, as described systematically by Mathes and Nahai, and by McCraw and coworkers. McLean and Buncke successfully used the omentum for reconstruction in the head and neck in 1972, and a little later McGregor and Jackson used a free transplant of a groin flap. This was used by Harii and coworkers, and later by Panje in the successful reconstruction in the head and neck area, although it has disadvantages: it is relatively thick and has only a short pedicle. The dorsalis pedis flap was also first described at that time, but poor healing at the donor site was frequent so that it was not widely used. Musculocutaneous flaps, like the latissimus dorsi flap, were also described for the first time in the early 1970s, and they were often used for reconstruction by microvascular surgeons.

Free flaps did not become established for several reasons, including difficulties in vessel anastomosis, so that better and more reliable tissue transfers were sought. By the end of the 1970s pedicled musculocutaneous flaps had been developed. The pectoralis major flap, developed by Ariyan in 1979, was especially popular. Three years earlier, Olivari had introduced the pedicled latissimus dorsi flap. With these flaps, reconstruction in the head and neck could be carried out in one operation in many cases. The limited length of the pedicle, the cosmetic limitations in the breast region with the pectoralis major flap, and the limited flexibility of this flap stimulated a renewed search for new transplants, so that free flaps were once again investigated.

At the end of the 1970s and the beginning of the 1980s many new reliable tissue transfers were developed. In 1978 a Chinese, Yang Guo-fan, and his colleagues used the radial forearm flap, for reconstruction of a severe neck burn. This flap was popularized outside China by Mühlbauer and coworkers in 1982. In 1979 Taylor presented the free iliac crest transplant for reconstruction of the mandible. Dos Santos in 1980 developed the scapular flap, and 2 years later a parascapular flap was presented by Nassif. There are now many free transplants and new ones are continually being developed.

Microvascular transplants are used in the head and neck area mainly for reconstruction of congenital defects and after trauma or excision of a tumor. They have clear advantages compared with pedicled musculocutaneous flaps in the reconstruction of the oropharynx, the hypopharynx, and the cervical esophagus. They have also proven themselves to be useful in the reconstruction of the contours of the face.

Free tissue transplantation is popular because a complex defect can be repaired in one session. They have extraordinary perfusion and heal well even in unfavorable situations, for example after radiation therapy and infection. Furthermore they do not have a bulky pedicle to disturb the transfer. The forearm flap has a long pedicle, which allows defects to be closed that are at a great distance from the anastamosed vessels. Another advantage is that the donor site is far away from the site demanding reconstruction. This avoids the problem of additional local scars. Also, scars, or changes in the skin due to radiation therapy, can hinder the introduction of a pedicled flap, so that it is sometimes impossible to adapt the skin over the pedicle, in which case the defect must be closed with a split skin graft.

Microvascular tissue transfers demand experience and knowledge that can be acquired only by special training. Satisfactory vessels must be found in the neck, which can be difficult after a prior operation or radiation therapy. Some vessels may already have been dissected, or the intima may be severely damaged by radiation, making anastomosis difficult and often leading to postoperative thrombi. If the vessel anastomosis is inadequate, the transplant may be completely lost. Unlike pedicled flaps, it is usually not possible to save part of the flap. Thus the surgeon who carries out free tissue transfers must be able to recognize complications early and be able to perform revision as needed.

The surgeon who works routinely with a surgical microscope has already acquired the basic skills required for microvascular surgery, but still needs thorough training in microvascular tissue transplantation.

References

Ariyan, S.: Further experiences with the pectoralis major myocutaneous flap for the immediate repair of a defect from excisions of head and neck cancers. Plast. reconstr. Surg. 64 (1979) 605–612

Daniel, R. K., G. I. Taylor: Distant transfer of an island flap by microvascular anastomoses. Plast. reconstr. Surg. 55 (1975) 177

Dos Santos, L. F.: The vascular anatomy and dissection of the free scapular flap. Plast. reconstr. Surg. 73 (1984) 59

Harii, K., K. Ohmori, S. Torii, F. Murakami, Y. Kasai, J. Sekiguchi, S. Ohmoni: Free groin skin flaps. Brit. J. plast. Surg. 28 (1975) 225

McCraw, J. B., L. T. Furlow: The dorsalis pedis arterialized flap: a clinical study. Plast. reconstr. Surg. 56 (1975) 13

McGregor, A., T. Jackson: The groin flap. Brit. J. plast. Surg. 25 (1972) 3

Mühlbauer, W., E. Herndl, W. Stock: The forearm flap. Plast. reconstr. Surg. 70 (1982) 336

Nassif, T. M., L. Vidal, J. L. Bovet, J. Baudet: The parascapular flap: A new cutaneous microsurgical free flap. Plast. reconstr. Surg. 69 (1982) 591–600

Olivari, N.: The latissimus flap. Brit. J. plast. Surg. 29 (1976) 126

Panje, W. R., C. J. Krause, J. Bardach et al.: Reconstruction of intraoral defects with the free groin flap. Arch.Otolaryngol. 103 (1977a) 78–83

Panje, W. R., C. J. Krause, J. Bardach: Microsurgical techniques in flap reconstruction. Laryngoscope 87 (1977b) 692–698

Seidenberg, B., S. Rosemak, E. S. Hurwitt: Immediate reconstruction of the cervical oesophagus by a revascularized isolated jejunal segment. Ann. Surg. 149 (1959) 162

Taylor, G. I., P. Townsend, R. Corlett: Superiority of the deep circumflex iliac vessels as the supply for the groin flaps. Plast. reconstr. Surg. 64 (1979) 595, 745

Yang, G., B. Chen, Y. Gao, X. Liu, J. Li, S. Jiang, S. He: Forearm free skin flap transplantation. Nat. med. J. China 61 (1981) 139

Basic Skills Required for Microvascular Surgery

Work under a microscope demands intense concentration coupled with slow and fine movements. Special experience and training are needed to learn the sequence of movements and to work with small instruments, because stitching under the microscope is very different from the macroscopic technique. The technique of microvascular surgery should be developed by practice using synthetic materials, blood vessels from slaughtered animals, such as pig spleen, or animal models.

Preliminary Exercises

Silicon tubes or surgical gloves serve as practice materials, for learning the basic concepts of microvascular surgery. The surgeon can accustom himself to visual relationships of size under the microscope, and to the use of the forceps and the needle holder. Vascular anastomosis on an animal, for example a rat, should not be attempted until experience has been gained with synthetic materials and blood vessels from slaughtered animals.

Forceps and needle holders are held like a pen (see Fig. 1.4). The middle finger supports the instrument from below, and the thumb and index finger rest on the instrument opposing each other. The instrument is moved by supination and pronation of the forearm resting on a flat surface, in order to reduce tremor, and by changing the grip, particularly of the index finger and thumb. Only the experienced microvascular surgeon should stitch without resting his forearm on a surface.

Even the removal of the suture from its package must be performed with care, because the needle may be bent or the suture ripped out of the needle. Therefore the needle should be removed carefully along its curvature, taking care that the suture does not snag on any part of the package. There are special suture packs that guarantee safe removal of the thread (see Fig. 18).

The needle is held with the needle holder one-third of its length from its blunt end, in such a way that the needle holder forms an angle of 90° with the needle.

Practice with Synthetic Materials

The first exercises may be carried out on surgical gloves, which can be stretched over an empty can and cut along markings. Practice cards are available (Fig. 1.1), which serve the same purpose.

The first exercise consists of sewing the cut edges back together, holding the instruments as described above. The needle is inserted about 1 mm from the cut edge, which is lifted with a forceps held in the left hand. The knot is made after piercing the opposite edge. The end of the suture must not be too long or too far from the point of insertion and it must not disappear from the field of vision.

The forceps, held in the left hand, grasps the suture about 2 cm from the point where the latter leaves the opposing edge and it is wound with two loops around the needle holder. The short end of the suture is then grasped by the needle holder and pulled through the loops. The knot must be pulled in the corresponding direction. Additionally, a single knot is made on top of the double knot in the opposite direction using the same procedure described above. The sutures are cut about 1 mm from the knots and lie, when knotted correctly, at about a 90° to the cut edge.

For the next step of the exercise a silicone tube (Fig. 1.2) with a 2-mm diameter is used. The forceps held in the left hand is inserted in the end of the tube with slightly opened limbs, so that it is possible to insert the needle into the wall of the tube exactly between the limbs. The resulting resistance facilitates the insertion of the needle. The needle can then be pushed through more easily when a forceps is pushed against the outer wall of the tube. A knot is made as described above, ensuring that there is no gap between the ends. Adaptation of the ends of the tubes is facilitated by using approximator clamps.

Before vessel anastomosis is attempted on animals, vessels from butchered animals can be used (pig's spleen and coronary arteries, chicken legs, etc.).

Exercises on Living Tissue

The abdominal aorta of the rat is particularly well suited for learning microvascular anastomosis (Fig. 1.3). The rat's abdomen is opened through a median incision from the xiphoid process to just above the bladder. Retractors are put in place, the animal's viscera are placed to the right and covered with a wet swab. This step provides good access to the retroperitoneum, where the major vessels (aorta and vena cava) are found. The aorta is carefully exposed, using blunt dissection, from the easily injured vena cava. Branches arising from the aorta must be li-

gated. When about 1.5–2 cm aorta is free, an approximator clip is applied to prevent retraction of the cut ends of the aorta. The clips can be brought so close together that the vessel ends almost touch.

The aorta is sutured as described above for the silicon tube. First angle sutures are laid at 150°, then another suture between the two angle sutures, and two further sutures between them, so that the front wall is closed with five stitches. When the sutures on the front wall are finished, the approximator clip is turned 180°, so that the back wall of the vessel now lies above. In this position the completed knots on the front wall can be checked from the inside through the still open back wall: the sutures must lie parallel, the distance between must be approximately equal, and all layers of the vessel wall, including the intima, should have been included in the suture. After the anastomosis is finished, the distal clip is opened first. If it appears that the suture is watertight, the proximal clip can be removed. If the suture is not tight, then another suture is placed at the gap.

Other suturing techniques, such as a continuous suture, and end-to-side anastomosis can also be practised on the rat aorta. A description of these techniques is found on pages 11–12, 14–15. Smaller vessels in the rat can also be anastomized, for example the carotid and femoral arteries (Mehdorn and Müller, 1987).

References

Acland, R. D.: Microsurgery. Practice Manual. Mosby, St. Louis 1980

Freys, S. M., Koob, E.: Ausbildung und Training in der Mikrochirurgie ohne Versuche am lebenden Tier. Handchirurgie 20, 11–16 1988

Govila, A.: A Simple Model on which to Practise Mikrosurgical Technique. Brit. J. Plast. Surg. 34, 486–487 1981

Mehdorn, H. M., G. H. Müller: Mikrochirurgische Übungen. Thieme, Stuttgart 1987

O'Brien, B. McC., W. A. Morrison: Reconstructive Microsurgery. Churchill-Livingstone, Edinburgh 1987

Pfander, A.: Zum Training der mikrochirurgischen Gefäß-Anastomose. Handchirurgie 12, 59–60 1980

Sućur, D., Konstantinović, P., Potparić, Z.: Fresh Chicken Leg: An Experimental Model for the Microsurgical Beginner. Brit. J. Plast. Surg. 34, 488–489 1981

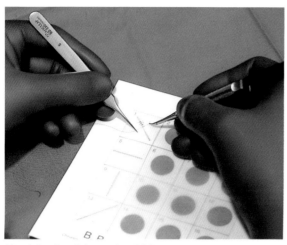

Fig. 1.1 Special preprinted foil cards are used to practice knot techniques. The foil is cut as marked and adapted using single sutures. Practice begins with a suture that is easy to knot, for example, 7–0 silk, progressing to 9–0 and 10–0 nylon suture.

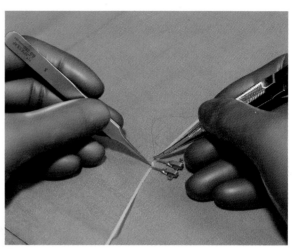

Fig. 1.2 Silicone tubing with a circumference of approximately 2 mm, held in a vascular clamp, is suitable as a model for end-to-end anastomosis, when the simple knotting technique has been mastered.

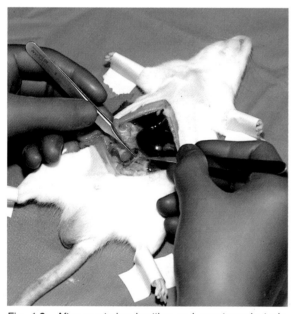

Fig. 1.3 After mastering knotting and anastomosis techniques on plastic materials, vessel anastomosis is practiced on an animal. The abdominal aorta of the rat is particularly well suited for this. The legal limitations and processes for acquiring approval for such a procedure should in all cases be respected.

Instruments

After the microforceps, the needle holder is one of the most important instruments in microvascular surgery. Formerly only two jeweler's forceps were used for microsurgery. The advantage of the needle holder is that the needle can be directed much more securely than with forceps. More difficult sewing techniques, such as backstitch, tension-stitch, or a stitch with the needle held at an acute angle, are then easier to carry out.

We prefer instruments for microvascular surgery that are shorter than 18 cm and weigh less than 30 g. They allow a fine action, but are stable enough to hold a 8–0 to 11–0 suture on a correspondingly small needle.

Needle Holder

We use a needle holder (Fig. 1.4a) with round handles, which can be turned through 45° to each side, allowing more mobility. Together with the curved working end, the jaws of the needle holder, the work range is extended to 180°. This makes the work much easier, when compared with the limited needle maneuverability available with a straight jeweler's forceps.

The needle holder is available with and without locking mechanism. We prefer micro needle holders that do not have a permanent locking mechanism, because the continual closing and

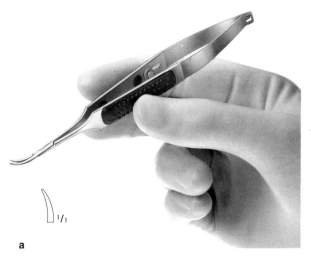
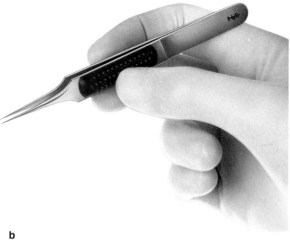

a

b

Fig. 1.4 a–b Microinstruments with the common round handle profile and different working ends. The instruments are held in the typical pen grip.
a Needle holder, b Forceps, c Scissors.

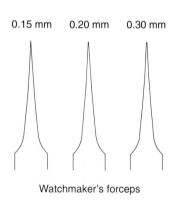

0.15 mm   0.20 mm   0.30 mm

Watchmaker's forceps

opening of the holder disturbs the fine motor activity. The locking mechanism facilitates placing and holding the suture, and is a relief for the nurse, who hands the instruments to the surgeon.

The handles of some instruments have a matte finish that improves the surgeon's grip and flexibility.

All instruments are self-opening. The spring systems are built so that they can be taken apart, to permit optimal cleaning of the moveable parts and joints.

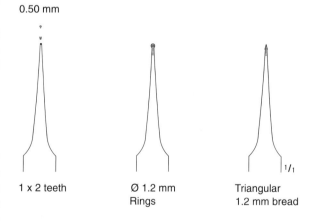

0.50 mm

1 x 2 teeth   Ø 1.2 mm Rings   Triangular 1.2 mm bread

Forceps

The range of microforceps (Fig. 1.4b) is continually being expanded and modified from the simple jeweler's forceps to suit the needs of the practitioner. The jeweler's forceps, fitted with a round-handle needle holder, still serves as the basic model. This instrument is simply making the work easier. The simple, straight jeweler's forceps has only a small area of contact at its working end, therefore profiles were developed with ring or triangular points, which have been used successfully for dissections. Plateau forceps, which allow the sutures to be securely held 2 to 3 mm from the tip, are available for better knotting.

Scissors

Microscissors (Fig. 1.4c) are available in straight and curved forms; the ends can be rounded or pointed. Scissors with rounded tips are particularly well suited for cutting the sutures, whereas scissors with pointed tips can be used for dissection. Button scissors were developed for perfo-

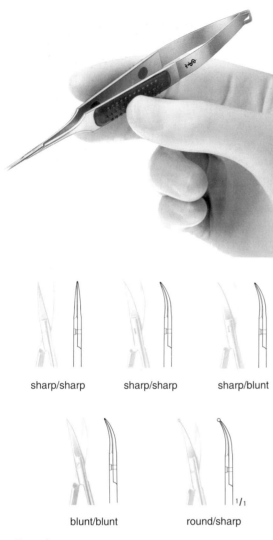

sharp/sharp   sharp/sharp   sharp/blunt

blunt/blunt   round/sharp

Fig. 1.**4c**

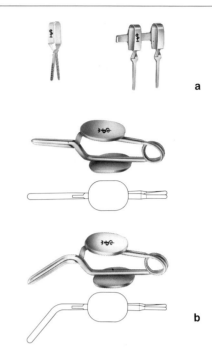

a

b

Fig. 1.**5**   Different vessel clips with varying closing pressures defined by the diameter of the vessel.
a Biemer clip, **b** Müller clip (alpha-principle).

rating the vessel wall in end-to-side anastomosis, and they allow precise dissection in the vessel lumen.

Vessel Clamps

Microclips are available in several models. We prefer Biemer clips (Fig. 1.5a) for vessels 1–2 mm in size; Acland clips (p. 58) can also be used. They have a frame that can take up the long ends of angle sutures during an end-to-end anastomosis; this is particularly helpful for the inexperienced. The closing pressure is optimally set at 25 g. Both types of clips are available as approximator clips—two clips on a bar. So-called approximator clips allow a reduction of tension at the ends of the vessels and make it possible to simultaneously adapt the vessels along their natu-

ral axes. However, they are usually too weak for vessels more than 3 mm in diameter. For that purpose the medium large-sized clamps are most suitable, which are designed according to the alpha-principle (Fig. 1.5b). This means that the arms close parallel, so that the pressure is spread evenly on the vessel wall. The clamps are particularly easy to put on, because they have microteeth. Another advantage is that the suture rarely falls into the clamp while a knot is being tied, because the spring end is closed. By exactly adjusting these clips to between 50 and 80 g, unnecessary damage to the vessels due to too much pressure is avoided.

For end-to-side anastomoses to the carotid artery or the jugular vein we use Satinski vessel clamps, which allow clamping of the area of the vessel to be sutured without dissection of the entire circumference of the vessel.

Care and Cleaning of Microinstruments

Microinstruments must be very carefully cleaned and cared for, because the fine working ends may be bent and the instruments rendered useless. They should first be cleaned with a fine brush under running water, to remove blood clots from the working ends and the microteeth. During the final cleaning in an ultrasound bath, fine instruments should not be mixed with larger ones. The locking mechanism must be regularly oiled to keep it mobile, and to allow unimpeded work. The instruments should be stored in a special rack so as to prevent damage, and in particular, to protect the working ends.

Microscope

The operating microscope may be either ceiling or floor mounted. A front lens with a focal length of from 200 to 250 mm is ideal for a relaxed working position in microvascular surgery. Direct coaxial lighting of the operational field by a light source built into the microscope carries a definite advantage over indirect lighting. The illumination of modern microscopes adapts smoothly to the magnification. It is set up in several axes, so that the lighting is even and free of shadows over the entire operational field.

For microsurgical tissue transplantation, magnification between 4 x and 10 x should be used. This is enough for good vision and for especially fine work, such as piercing the vessel wall with the needle. Microscopes with zoom lenses are ideal. The smooth adaptation to the operative field permits accurate work without fatigue. Furthermore it is not necessary to lay down instruments in order to change the magnification.

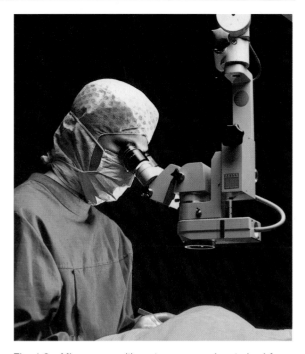

Fig. 1.6   Microscope with motor zoom and motorized focus makes the microsurgical procedures easier. Maneuverable arms allow the surgeon to work without tiring and to achieve optimal adjustment to the operating field. Operating microscope OPMI MD with tiltable binocular tubes 0–60°.

Tiltable binocular tubes (60° or 180°) (Figs 1.6, 1.7) that carry the eyepieces allow the surgeon to choose a comfortable seated posture and

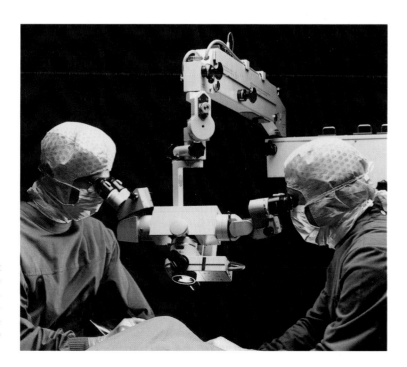

Fig. 1.7   A special beam splitter makes it possibe for both surgeons to have binocular visual field, guaranteeing optimal assistance, particularly during learning of vessel anastomosis. Operating microscope OPMI MD with beam splitter L/1 and two tiltable binocular tubes 0–180°.

position of the head. The eyepieces should be adjusted exactly according to the distance between the eyes. For those who wear glasses, the eyepieces should be adjusted with their rubber adapters, in order to ensure the same panoramic vision that is possible without glasses. During learning of vessel anastomosis under the guidance of an experienced microvascular surgeon, special stereo beam splitters are available that allow a binocular vision for both surgeons and optimal spatial orientation for the assistant.

After the basic position is established the arm of the microscope is locked in place. At this point the optical adjustment is carried out; the receptor vessel is brought into focus at the highest magnification, and from the magnification (ca. 25 x) is then zoomed back to a working magnification (ca. 4 x to 6 x), to provide an optimal depth of sharp focus.

A 4 x to 6 x magnification is sufficient for dissection of a vessel; but for anastomosis a higher magnification is needed. Then sutures are made under a lower magnification, because a broad depth of field is needed to enable the end of the thread to be found.

Sterile microscope covers are available for work in an operating room to protect against blood, etc. Detachable sterile rubber knobs, which offer both less protection and sterility, are preferred by some surgeons.

Suture Materials

In the last 10 years the choice of materials for microvascular surgery has increased greatly. Suture material can be differentiated according to the following criteria:

- Type of suture, material, and color
- Thickness of suture
- Length of suture
- Type of needle, its end, shape, and weight
- Size of needle

Microsuture material is offered by several manufacturers in a thickness of 7–0 to 12–0. For microvascular surgery, 8–0 to 10–0 sutures have proven optimal (Fig. 1.8). The choice of material must depend on its characteristics. There are absorbable and nonabsorbable suture materials. Until now absorbable sutures have rarely been indicated for microvascular surgery. Even nonabsorbable sutures are subject to dissolution but this can take years (polyamide, nylon). Sutures may be made from silk, nylon, polypropylene, polyamide, or polyester. Polyfilament and monofilament sutures are available. The polyfilament suture, as is known from general surgery, provides a more stable knot than the monofilament, but is hardly used because of its traumatizing effects on the vessel wall when the suture is pulled through.

No less important than the mechanical qualities of the suture are its visual characteristics. Strongly colored and highly contrasting sutures are preferable to pale ones, particularly at higher magnifications and in difficult lighting situations. Black sutures are much easier to recognize under the microscope than green, blue, or violet. Because nylon sutures are colored by mixing with particles of ink, not only is the intensity of contrast dependent on the quantity of the dye but also the mechanical quality of the sutures. The strength and the adaptation to knotting is reduced when the suture is dyed, and its elasticity and stability change. The process of sterilization can also influence the mechanical qualities. Gamma-ray sterilization reduces the suture's tensile strength.

The strength of a suture is determined by its diameter. A 10–0 suture has less than a quarter of the diameter of a 9–0 suture, so that its resistance to breakage is reduced. This plays a role in special sewing techniques, such as a continuous suture. The suture is particularly easily damaged through direct contact with the instruments; in particular, it can be damaged in the process of being knotted with a watchmaker's forceps and a needle holder. A heavier suture would naturally be less damaged by such a manipulation than a thinner one. It is usual in microvascular surgery, however, to use as fine a suture as possible, in order to introduce the least amount of foreign material into the body.

In addition to the material and thickness of the suture, the length also plays an important role. Obviously it is up to the surgeon to shorten the suture to a length that he or she feels comfortable with–shorter sutures usually make vessel suture easier. Even double-ended sutures are available, but we believe there is no place for them, except possibly for open or continuous sutures in order to save time. The optimal suture length depends on the chosen technique. Long sutures can also be used for interrupted sutures, whereas shorter sutures are advantageous in continuous suture techniques. Long sutures have proven to be useful in open prelaid sutures. Finally, length is also important if the suturing is done on the surface or deeper levels.

It is simple to chose the needles for small vessels in microsurgery. The size of the needle should be between 4 and 6 mm. It should be three-eighths of a circle and between 70 and 150 μm thick.

Another important characteristic is the cutting characteristic of the needle. Hard steel needles have a better cutting edge with a long, sharp point and do not bend so easily. They also stay sharp longer, but are not so easy to thread. Soft needles with short points are common, but should be avoided. The shinier a needle appears under the microscope, the sharper and more stable it is.

The shape of the needle varies: there are round, oval, or flattened forms. Asymmetric shapes are said to be easier to grasp with the needle holder. As soon as the needle holder closes, the needle slides into the correct position according to its beveling. A second instrument is usually necessary for round needles. Time can be saved by selecting the appropriate materials in the first place.

The way the suture is attached to the needle varies from manufacturer to manufacturer. The union must be carefully made to avoid large insertion holes as the needle passes through the tissue, leading to more bleeding. The needle usually has a flattened notch, the suture is laid in the notch and the edges are pressed together. Sutures can also be inserted in predrilled needles (laser drilling) and can be stabilized by simple crushing or gluing. Further developments in this area may be expected.

The packaging is usually characteristic of a particular manufacturer. Double packaging is necessary to ensure sterility. Possible damage to the suture or needle should be ascertained when the first package is opened. The needle must be kept in a protected setting and should be simple to remove, that is, it should be either easily visible when inserted into a small soft needle holder (Fig. 1.8) or it should be kept in an obvious, easy-to-recognize open space in a needle holder. The first option usually comes with a loose-lying suture, the second generally has sutures wound around it.

Long packs are ideal for the removal of two or more sutures: they are already offered by various companies for practice and teaching purposes. The removal process in this case is particularly protective because the sutures lie stretched out lengthwise between two foam rubber pads. The needles lie either free or are easily removed from the foam rubber pads. In practice, however,

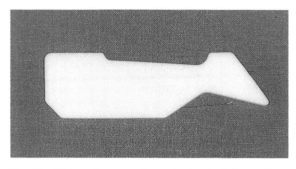

Fig. 1.8 The most commonly used suture is 9–0 on a 5-mm needle in packing specially designed for microsutures. The needle is inserted into a synthetic cushion so that it can be removed by the undamaged needle holder.

these multipacks are not cost effective because they usually cannot be resterilized. A selection with two sutures in each is ideal for microvascular surgery. We prefer 8–0 to 9–0 suture material with a needle between 5 and 6 mm. Black nylon has proven to be the best.

Suture and Anastomosis Technique

Suture Technique
(Figs. 1.9–1.19)

The knots are always tied under the microscope using instruments, normally a needle holder and microforceps. Plateau forceps are particularly good, because they grasp the suture securely and do little harm to its surface. The suture is more often damaged with jeweler's forceps, and can later tear at that spot.

In principle only standard knots should be used which must be firm and secure. Knots should not be made under tension, so that the ends of the vessels must be optimally approximated. The suture is tied at an exact right angle to the line of anastomosis. The ends of the sutures must be pulled parallel to the axis of the vessel. The second knot is turned on a 180° axis and the double knot completed. If the same exact knotting technique is used for the interrupted sutures and all these procedures are followed, the ends of the sutures will run exactly parallel to the vessel. This has the great advantage that if necessary, restitching between two knots is easily possible. It is a basic principle of surgery that tidy work is often functionally better.

In contrast to macrosurgery, where a suture may be knotted from six to eight times by hand to achieve security, this is not permissible in mi-

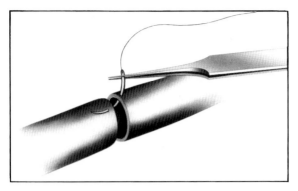

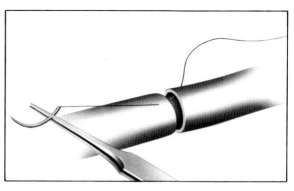

Fig. 1.**9** Single suture. The needle is inserted through several wall layers of the donor and receptor vessels close to the vessel ends with a rotating movement that corresponds to the curve of the needle.

Fig. 1.**10**   The suture is pulled through by gripping the needle, because pulling the suture directly would damage it.

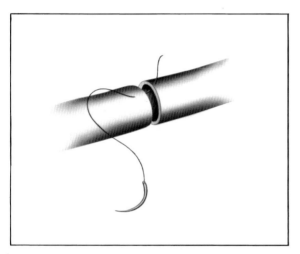

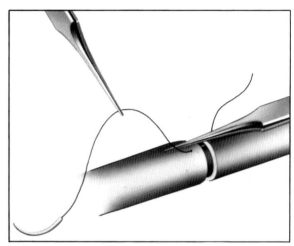

Fig. 1.**11**   After the suture is pulled through until only a short end remains, the needle is parked within the field of vision, for example, by inserting it into a muscle.

Fig. 1.**12**   The suture is grasped by the left-hand forceps about 1.5–2 cm from the point where it leaves the vessel and wound to the right around the right-hand forceps (needle holder) (F).

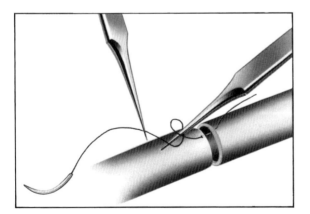

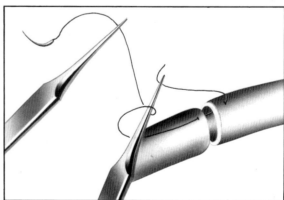

Fig. 1.**13**   The right-hand forceps continues the movement.

Fig. 1.**14** ·   The right-hand forceps grasps the short end of the suture and both forceps pull in opposite directions along the line of the blood vessel, to complete the first knot.

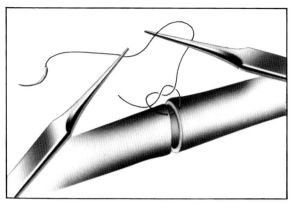

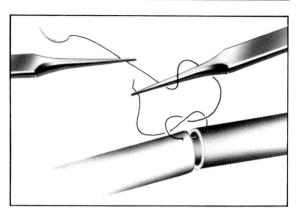

Fig. 1.15   To tie an opposing knot the left-hand forceps takes the suture and winds it to the left around the right-hand forceps, completing the movement.

Fig. 1.16   The right-hand forceps grasps the short end of the suture and both forceps pull in opposite directions along the line of the blood vessel, to complete the second knot.

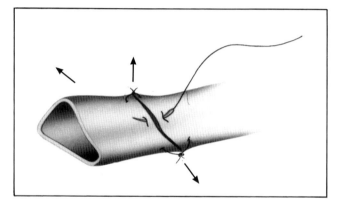

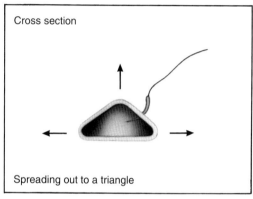

Fig. 1.17   For interrupted sutures the vessel can be opened up in the shape of a triangle, to make the technique easier and to ensure that the front wall is not sewn to the back wall.

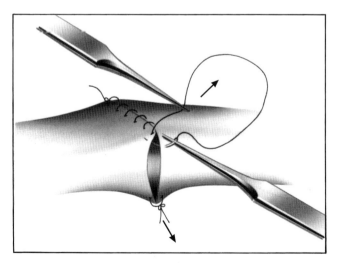

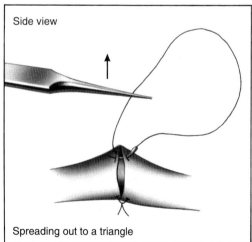

Fig. 1.18   The vessel is pulled into triangular shape during a continuous suture also, by traction on the suture about 1 cm from the needle hole. This step demands great care to prevent injury to the suture.

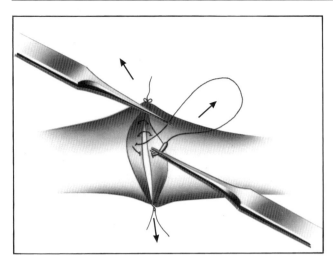 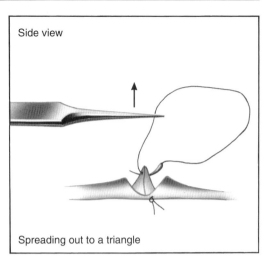

Side view

Spreading out to a triangle

Fig. 1.19   The back wall of the vessel can be sewn in a similar way to that of the front wall, through the still open front wall. The angle sutures can be fixed in a frame, in a small clamp, or by sewing them to neighboring tissue.

crosurgery. Thus accurate standard knots must be tied with the help of instruments to ensure a high degree of firmness after two or three knots.

Anastomosis Technique

Different techniques are available for end-to-end and end-to-side anastomosis. We have standardized four basic techniques, with which all situations encountered in reconstructive microvascular surgery can be mastered.

The limited range of movement within the surgical field and the restricted view make special suture techniques necessary. For the beginner, interrupted sutures are generally more reliable than continuous ones. In the course of standardizing the techniques we observed that a flexing hand movement is easier to achieve than a stretching one. Rows of sutures laid towards the surgeon are easier to place than those in the opposite direction. Assistance is rarely feasible and surgery must be performed, with either hand capable of holding the microinstruments.

End-to-End Anastomosis
with Interrupted Sutures
(Figs. 1.20–1.25)

The most common anastomosis, used especially for arteries, is end-to-end anastomosis. The line of anastomosis is ideally performed while the vessel axis is at an angle of 45°. The most comfortable position of the hand in relation to the direction of suturing is, however, often impossible

to find because of the anatomical situation. Both ends of the vessels are approximated. Suturing begins with a lower angle suture then a second angle suture is placed above, approximately at 160–170° on the other side. Another suture is then placed in the middle between the two angle sutures. The forceps can be placed in the vessel lumen with its blades slightly opened, so as to lift the wall of the vessel slightly and make the insertion of the needle easier. However, the intima must not be injured. Two more sutures are made between each of the three already present. The vessel is then turned—this is made particularly simple by the use of Biemer–Müller approximator clips. The row of sutures on the front wall is first inspected through the still open back wall of the vessel. The sutures should lie parallel and have approximately equal breadth of stitch. In particular, all layers must be included in the suture. The suture should never run between the intima and media, because blood could enter at that point and strip the intima. The back wall is closed in the same way as the front, ensuring that the latter is not inadvertently included in a stitch, because a final inspection of the sutures is no longer possible.

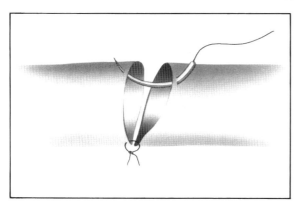

Fig. 1.**20** After placing the lower angle suture, the upper suture is made on the opposite side at an angle of about 160–170° (measuring from the diameter of the vessel in a downward direction), so that the front wall is shortened in relation to the back wall.

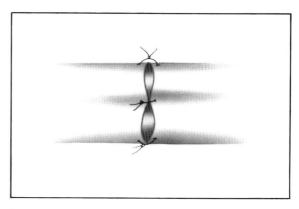

Fig. 1.**21** The next suture is made in the middle between the two angle sutures.

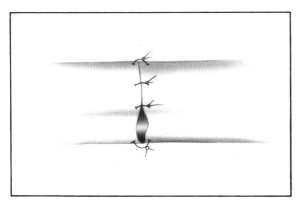

Fig. 1.**22** Two further sutures are made between the middle and angle sutures.

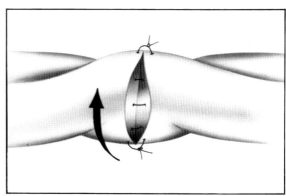

Fig. 1.**23** The vessel is rotated to allow inspection of the already completed suture line of the front wall from the vessel lumen.

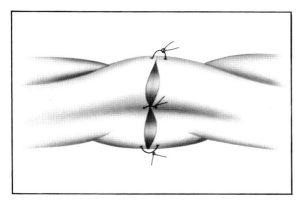

Fig. 1.**24** Suture in the middle of the back wall.

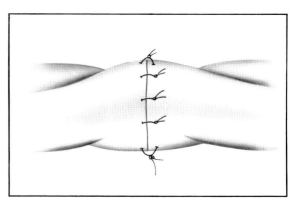

Fig. 1.**25** Further sutures between the middle and angle sutures.

*End-to-End Anastomosis
with a Continuous Suture*
(Figs. 1.26–1.31)

A continuous suture is carried out from the outside, with the vessel ends in approximator clips, so that the vessel can be turned. If this is not the case, the back wall is sewn from the inside of the vessel. In microvascular surgery, unlike other vascular surgery, end-to-end suture using a continuous technique is not as suitable for arteries as for veins. Sutures have to be carefully knotted in thinly walled veins, in order to avoid the danger of stenosis. Therefore, we try to lay the last suture only after the clips have been removed; the area of anastomosis expands in the process. At the least, we open the distal vessel clip, which usually causes a backflow of venous blood and makes it possible to put controlled pressure on

the anastomosis when the last knot is tied. If the vessel cannot be turned, the back wall is first sewn through the still open front wall, while angle sutures are placed first. Then another suture next to the angle sutures is placed, while the needle is not cut off the thread in order to enable continuous suturing. The needle is once again inserted through the vessel wall, from the outside in, the suture is grasped by the forceps about 2 cm from the vessel, and pulled so that the back wall of both vessel ends can be drawn through the still open front wall. Next both vessel walls are pierced close to the cut edge, and the suture is again grasped by the forceps and pulled. When the second angle suture is reached the needle is passed through the vessel wall from the inside and the end of the suture is knotted to the long end of the angle suture. Then the front wall can be continuously sutured in the usual way.

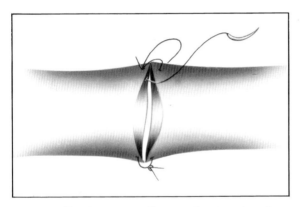

Fig. 1.26   After the upper and lower angle sutures have been made, the needle is passed from the outside to the inside near the upper angle suture.

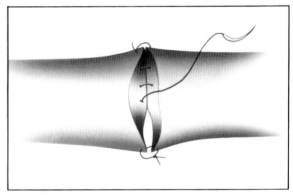

Fig. 1.27   The continuous suture of the back wall sewn through the open front wall is carried out as in Figure 1.19.

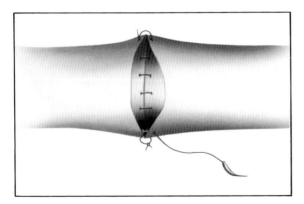

Fig. 1.28   When the lower angle suture is reached the needle is passed from the inside to the outside.

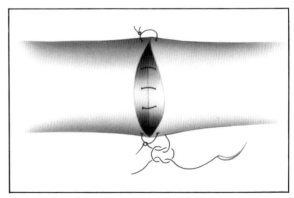

Fig. 1.29   Knotting the suture with the long end to the angle suture. If it is drawn too tightly, the back wall can shorten.

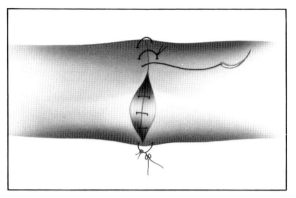

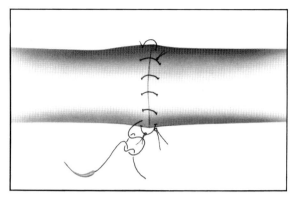

Fig. 1.**30** Suturing of the front wall begins close to the upper angle suture and is carried out as in figure 1.**18**.

Fig. 1.**31** When the lower angle suture is reached the suture is tied to the long end of the angle suture.

End-to-Side Anastomosis
with Interrupted Sutures
(Figs. 1.**32**–1.**37**)

End-to-side anastomosis differs from end-to-end anastomosis in the sequence the sutures are

made: the third and fourth sutures are each placed close to the angle sutures. The back wall is exposed by turning the vessel, as already described, and closed with interrupted sutures in the same way. End-to-side anastomosis with interrupted sutures is mainly used for arteries.

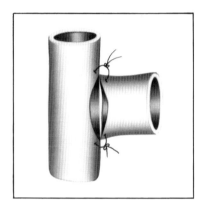

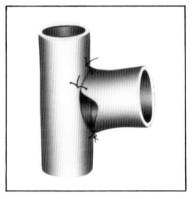

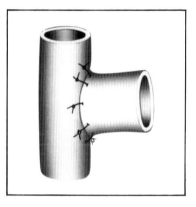

Fig. 1.**32** After creating an opening of sufficient size in the receptor vessel, the upper and lower angle sutures are placed.

Fig. 1.**33** Unlike an end to end anastomosis, the next suture placed next to the angle sutures.

Fig. 1.**34** Suture in the middle of the front wall.

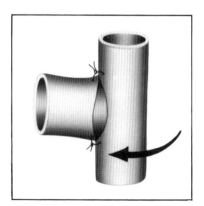

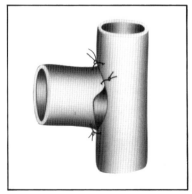

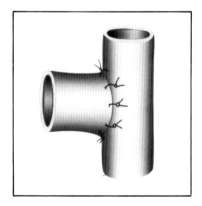

Fig. 1.**35** Turning the vessel.

Fig. 1.**36** Two further sutures are placed close to the angle sutures.

Fig. 1.**37** The last suture is made in the middle of the back wall.

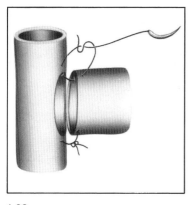

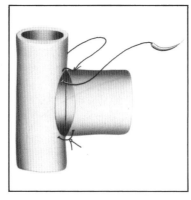

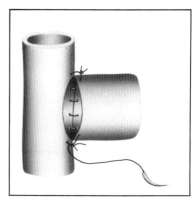

1.38

1.39

1.40

Fig. 1.38   Upper and lower angle sutures.

Fig. 1.39   A second knot for the continuous suture is made close to the upper angle suture.

Fig. 1.40   Continuous suturing of the back wall is carried out as shown in Figure 1.19 through the still open front wall. The suture is passed from the inside to the outside and knotted to the lower angle suture.

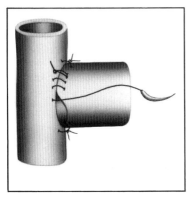

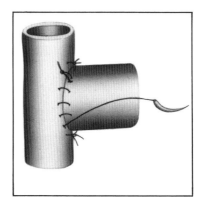

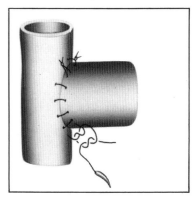

1.41

1.42

1.43

Fig. 1.41   Suturing of the front wall begins close to the upper angle suture, initially from the outside to the inside, then from the inside to the outside.

Fig. 1.42   The running suture is continued to the lower angle suture.

Fig. 1.43   Knotting of the suture to the long end of the angle suture.

End-to-Side Anastomosis with a Continuous Suture
(Figs. 1.38–1.43)

In principle, there is no difference between the procedure for a continuous suture of an end-to-side anastomosis and that for an end-to-end anastomosis. After the angle sutures have been placed, the continuous suture is begun on the back wall, stitching from the outside in. At the end of the row the thread passes from the inside out and is knotted to the lower angle suture, as already described for continuous end-to-end anastomosis. The front wall is sewn similarly with a continuous everting suture from the outside. End-to-side anastomosis with a continuous suture is used mainly for veins.

Different Types of Tissue and their Blood Supplies

The loss of specific tissue due to trauma, tumor resection, radiation treatment, etc., demands reconstruction with tissue that most closely resembles the lost tissue. Microvascular tissue transplantation is ideal for this process because tissue, such as skin, muscle, and bone from distant parts of the body can be used. For example, for reconstruction of the oral cavity and the oropharynx, a thin fasciocutaneous flap or a segment of small intestine can be used; a multiple defect with the loss of part of the mandible can be repaired with a musculocutaneous or an osteocutaneous transplant. In choosing the appropriate tissue it is preferable that the donor site lie far from the head and neck region. Thus it is possible to operate simultaneously in the donor and receptor sites. This is possible in all of the flaps discussed below except for the scapular and parascapular flaps.

Clinically, the following transplants have proven to be useful for the head and neck:

- Free cutaneous or fasciocutaneous flaps:
  - Forearm flap
  - Dorsalis pedis flap
  - Scapular and parascapular flaps

- Free muscle and/or musculocutaneous flaps:
  - Latissimus dorsi flaps
  - Rectus abdominis flaps

- Free bone transplants, osteocutaneous, and osteomyocutaneous flaps:
  - Iliac crest
  - Scapular and parascapular flaps

- Jejunum and omentum

McGregor and Morgan (1973) defined two different kinds of pedicled flap: axial pattern (Fig. 1.44) and random pattern (Fig. 1.45). The first flap has an anatomically defined vascular system, which stretches along its axis; the second does not. Many axial pattern flaps are well suited for microvascular tissue transplantation. The first flaps so defined were the deltopectoral, hypogastric, and groin flaps.

Every tissue that has a closed arteriovenous circulation is suitable for use as a free transplant. The following prerequisites must be fulfilled by tissue to be transplanted in clinical practice:

- The pedicle that supplies the tissue to be transplanted must consist of at least one ar-

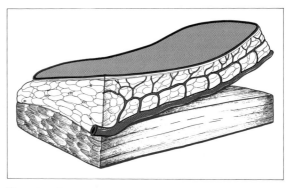

Fig. 1.**44**   The axial pattern flap has an anatomically defined arteriovenous system, which runs along the length of the axis of the flap. It is suitable for free tissue transfer provided that the diameter of the vessel is large enough for microvascular anastomosis (more than 0.8 mm).

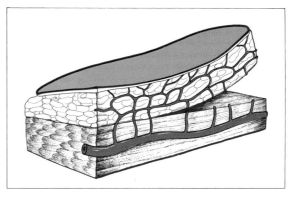

Fig. 1.**45**   The random pattern flap receives its blood supply from small perforator vessels that arise from a vessel in deeper lying tissue. This flap can be used for advancement, rotation, or transposition flaps, but is unsuitable for free tissue transfer.

tery and one, or preferably, two veins; they must have a sufficient diameter (greater than 0.8 mm) to be used for microvascular anastomosis

- The vessels must have enough branches to supply the entire flap
- The anatomical variation in the course of the vessel should be minimal
- Dysfunction at the donor site should be minimal

The skin is supplied by two different vascular systems, direct cutaneous arteries, and musculocutaneous arteries. The latter are small vessels that arise from a larger segmental muscle artery, spread fan-like into the skin, and supply it and the muscle. An example of this type of blood

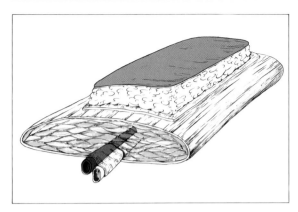

Fig. 1.**46** The myocutaneous flap consists of musculature with the overlying skin. The main vessel axis runs in the muscle. Perforator vessels run from it through the muscle to the skin above. If skin is needed for reconstruction it can be removed with the underlying muscle. It is usually possible, however, to remove a section of muscle which is thinner than the skin that lies above it.

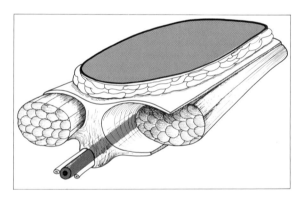

Fig. 1.**47** The fasciocutaneous flap, for example the forearm flap, includes the underlying fascia. The pedicle runs in the intermuscular fascia in a plane deeper than the actual skin flap; the distance can be as much as 3 cm with an forearm flap. The skin area is supplied by small perforator vessels arising from the main pedicle.

supply is seen in the latissimus dorsi flap (Fig. 1.**46**).

Cutaneous arteries, as seen in the forearm flap (Fig. 1.**47**), run above the deep fascia to perfuse larger skin areas. The venous drainage passes through a superficial and a deep venous system, which are separated from each other by a layer of subcutaneous fat tissue. The superficial venous system is a network of vessels that converge into larger veins and that have no relation to the arteries in their course. The deep venous system is arranged in the form of a rope ladder accompanying the arteries (venae comitantes).

This anatomical knowledge is important in planning a flap and its dissection. The dissection of a flap may not extend beyond the limits of its pedicle, because otherwise necrotic edges may develop. There are exact descriptions of almost every flap in the literature, based on anatomical studies of their blood supply.

References

Bakamjian, V. Y.: A two-stage method for pharyngoesophageal reconstruction with a primary pectoral skin flap. Plast. reconstr. Surg. 36 (1965) 173–184

McCraw, J. B., P. G. Arnold: McCraw and Arnold's Atlas of Muscle and Musculocutaneous Flaps. Hampton Press, Norfolk/Va. 1986

Mc Gregor, I. A., I. T. Jackson: The groin flap. Brit. J. plast. Surg. 25 (1972) 3–16

Mc Gregor, I., G. Morgan: Axial and random pattern flaps. Brit. J. plast. Surg. 26 (1973) 202–213

Rollin, K. D., H. B. Williams: The free transfer of skin flaps by microvascular anastomoses. An experimental study and a reappraisal. Plast. reconstr. Surg. 52 (1973) 16–31

Shaw, D. T., R. L. Payne: One stage tubed abdominal flaps. Surg. Gynecol. Obstet. 83 (1946) 205–209

Smith, P. J.: The vascular basis of axial pattern flaps. Brit. J. plast. Surg. 26 (1973) 150

Strauch, B., H-L Yu: Atlas of microvascular surgery. Thieme Medical Publishers, New York (1993)

Taylor, G. I., K. D. Rollin: The anatomy of several free flap donor sites. Plast. reconstr. Surg. 56 (1975) 243–253

Timmons, M. J.: Landmarks in the anatomical study of the blood supply of the skin. Brit. J. plast. Surg. 38 (1985) 197–202

2 Technique of Flap Removal

Forearm Flap

The forearm flap was first developed by Yang Guofan and his coworkers in China in 1978. For this reason it is referred to as the Chinese flap in the American literature. Mühlbauer and colleagues popularized the method outside China.

The flap is a fasciocutaneous graft that is particularly well suited to the reconstruction of superficial defects in the entire head and neck region. The graft can be used for reconstruction of the pharynx and oral cavity as well as the external head and neck because it can be so well modeled. The graft can be harvested at the same time as the tumor is removed. The patient can be quickly remobilized because the defect of the forearm does not impair function.

The graft consists of a section of skin with its underlying fascia, of variable size, taken from the volar surface of the forearm. It is also possible to remove the graft with a segment of the radius for use as an osteocutaneous transplant, but this is not common in the head and neck because more suitable transplants are available for reconstruction of the mandible.

Either the radial or the ulnar artery can be used to nourish the forearm flap. Some authors describe the graft based on the ulnar artery, and prefer it to the radial forearm graft, but the dissection is more difficult than that of the radial artery, which takes a more regular course.

Vascular Anatomy

The radial artery (Fig. 2.1) lies in a neurovascular bundle together with the superficial branch of the radial nerve lying laterally. The nerve separates from the vessels in the distal third of the forearm and passes the brachioradialis tendon on its way to the back of the hand. The radial artery lies superficially along the entire length of the forearm, between the brachioradialis and

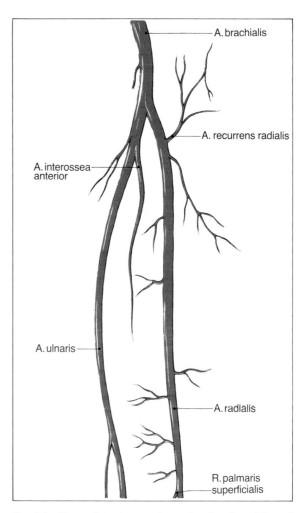

Fig. 2.1 The radial artery continues the direction of flow of the brachial artery, from which the ulnar artery arises at the elbow. The interosseous artery branches off from the ulnar artery. The superficial palmar branches arise near the carpal ligaments. Along the entire length of the vessel branches arise at regular intervals from the skin and musculature.

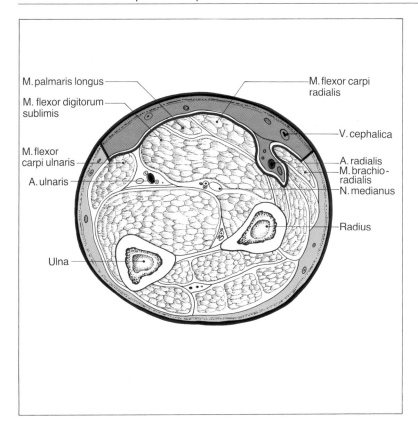

M. palmaris longus

M. flexor digitorum sublimis

M. flexor carpi ulnaris

A. ulnaris

Ulna

M. flexor carpi radialis

V. cephalica

A. radialis
M. brachio-radialis
N. medianus

Radius

Fig. 2.**2**   Cross section through the distal forearm. The neurovascular bundle (radial artery, venae comitantes and the superficial branch of the radial nerve) lies in the intermuscular fascia between the flexor carpi radialis and the brachioradialis muscles.

pronator teres muscles in the proximal third, and between the brachioradialis and flexor carpi radialis muscles or ligaments in the distal two-thirds (Figs. 2.**2**, 2.**3**).

After the radial recurrent artery has branched off, no large vessels leave the radial artery until the superficial palmar branch. The radial artery connects with the ulnar artery via the palmar arch. It supplies the entire volar and a part of the dorsolateral forearm skin through cutaneous vessel branches, which are more thickly ramified distally than proximally. The flap drains through the veins accompanying the radial artery as well as through superficial veins. The basilic, cephalic, and median veins are all available subcutaneous veins. The median vein is, however, usually too small and unsafe for vessel anastomosis, and the basilic vein lies too far medially so that only the cephalic or comitantes venae are suitable for venous drainage. There are connections between the superficial veins and venae and comitantes veins, so that it does not make much difference which venous system is used for the anastomosis, but we prefer the deeper system.

Flap Planning

The flap can be harvested distally (Fig. 2.**4a**) or proximally (Fig. 2.**4b**); it is even possible to include the entire volar surface of the forearm. The flap increases in thickness from the distal to the proximal end because of the increase in subcutaneous fat tissue, but the pedicle becomes shorter. In the proximal forearm the radial artery often lies in a deep intermuscular fascia, which makes dissection of the flap more difficult (Fig. 2.**4c**). A flap removed from a distal site leaves a defect, with many tendons exposed, in contrast to one taken from the middle or proximal region, which exposes muscle bellies.

Before the dissection begins, the site and size of the graft must be determined, taking into account retraction of approximately one-quarter in size. The size is determined by how thick and how large the flap should be, what length pedicle is required, and whether or not hair is present. Before the dissection begins, the flap and the course of the radial artery are marked out (Fig. 2.**5**).

Prior to harvesting the flap it is necessary to determine whether the entire hand can be supplied by the ulnar artery using Allen's test, Doppler sonography, pulsoxymetry, or angiography. In Allen's test the patient is asked to open and close the fist ten times, and after the tenth time to keep it closed. The radial and ulnar arteries are compressed and the patient opens the fist, whereby the ulnar artery is then released. If the entire capillary system of the hand rapidly refils, then the ulnar artery can irrigate the whole hand. In doubtful cases the radial artery can be bridged with a vein graft, but this is rarely necessary. The flap should be taken from the nondominant hand.

Angiography is rarely needed.

Flap Elevation

We do not use a tourniquet during dissection of the flap to ensure that the perfusion can be observed throughout the flap elevation. After making an S-shaped incision from a point distal to the elbow to the proximal edge of the flap, the forearm fascia is split, during which attention should be paid to superficial veins, which can usually be coagulated with bipolar forceps. The flexor carpi and the brachioradialis muscles are exposed and the bellies separated by cutting the intermuscular fascia (Fig. 2.6), which appears a white band lying between the two muscles. At this point small arteries, usually accompanied by two veins, signal the proximity of the pedicle of the radial artery with the venae comitantes lying between the two muscle bodies on the fascia of the flexor digitorum superficialis muscle.

The pedicle is dissected only up to the point where it remains bound by the fascia. The primary exposure of the pedicle allows assessment of whether the venae comitantes of the radial artery are of sufficient circumference to permit microvascular anastomosis. If so the dissection of a superficial vein is unnecessary. If the veins appear too small, however, a superficial vein can be included in the dissection. On a distal flap the cephalic vein lies too far laterally, so a middle superficial vein should be used. On a middle or proximal flap the cephalic vein, which lies radial to the radial artery over the superficial fascia on the brachioradialis muscle, is preferably used. The accompanying veins are indeed thinner than the radial artery, but if the artery and its accompanying veins are followed to the elbow a venous plexus is found as the venae comitantes unite with the deep vein system of the brachial

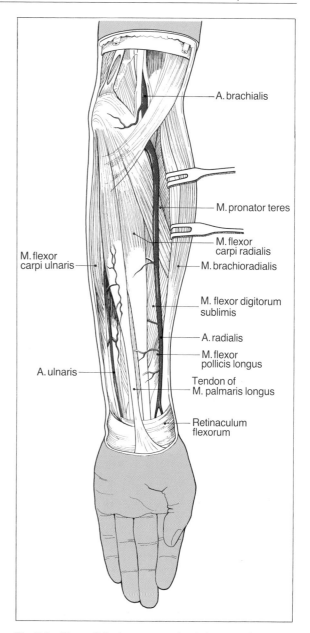

Fig. 2.3   The radial artery passes deeply between the pronator teres muscle and the brachioradialis muscle, then superficially between the tendons of the flexor carpi radialis and brachioradialis muscles towards the wrist. The muscle bellies lie mainly in the proximal region of the forearm, and pass distally into their respective tendons.

veins. A short segment of this venous plexus can be used as a connecting vessel. Its circumference, usually over 2 mm, is clearly larger than the venae comitantes. After the flap has been elevated, the entire pedicle is dissected with it proximally and fully separated from the fascia of the flexor digitorum superficialis muscle, on which it lies.

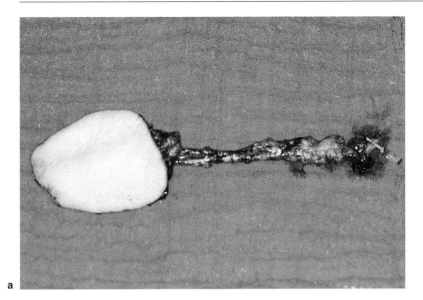

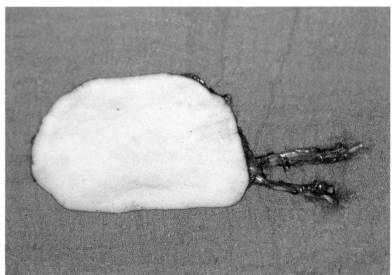

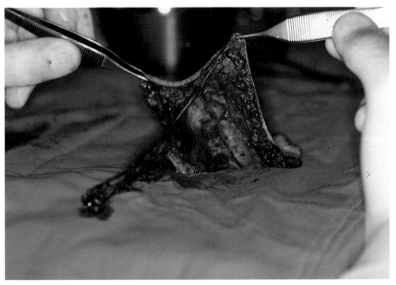

Fig. 2.4   Radial forearm flap. **a** Small flap from a distal site. **b** A larger flap from the middle third, with both the radial artery and accompanying veins; in **b** the cephalic vein is included in the dissection. **c** At a proximal site, the vessel can run in a deep intermuscular fascia, which makes the dissection much more difficult.

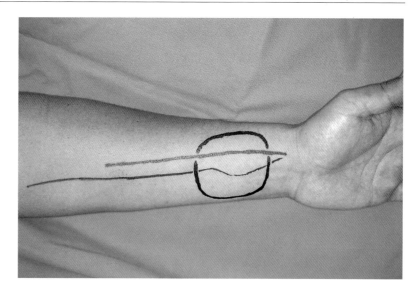

Fig. 2.**5** Planning the flap on the volar forearm. The small distal flap is thin, and consequently easily modeled, and has a long pedicle.

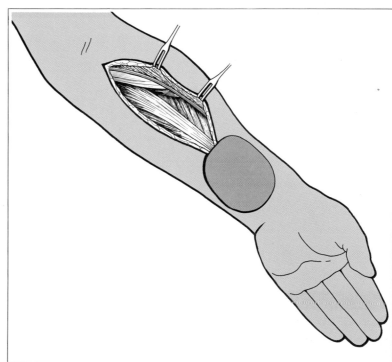

Fig. 2.**6** The first operative step is to expose the pedicle. In the proximal or middle third of the forearm, this requires that the antebrachial fascia between the flexor carpi radialis and the brachioradialis muscles be cut. The radial artery is covered by the brachioradialis muscle, which must be retracted laterally to expose the pedicle. Several vessels that enter the muscle must be cut during the dissection of the pedicle.

Next, the edges of the flap are incised (Fig. 2.7), cutting through the fascia on the ulnar edge of the flexor digitorum sublimis. The flap together with the fascia is dissected from the ulnar towards the radial border. If the dissection is carried out in the middle third of the forearm it should be remembered that this is the region in which the muscle bellies give off their tendons (flexor digitorum sublimis, palmaris longus, and flexor carpi radialis muscles). The dissection over the tendons should be done very carefully, in order not to injure the paratenon. In the distal region attention must be paid to the ulnar artery during dissection because it may follow an atypical course. It can run over the flexor digitorum sublimis muscle medially up to the ulnar edge of the tendon of the flexor carpi radialis and be injured there. It is important to protect the ulnar artery, which, in contrast to the radial artery, sometimes runs superficially and irregularly.

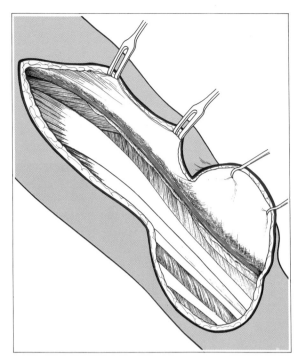

Fig. 2.**7**   After incising around the edge of the flap the fascia of the flexor digitorum muscle is cut. The flap is dissected with the muscle fascia from medial to lateral. It is carefully separated from the underlying muscles and tendons in order to avoid injury to the paratenon. After the pedicle has been lifted from the flexor digitorum superficialis or flexor pollicis longus muscle, it must be dissected away from the tendon of the brachioradialis muscle. It is important to pay attention to the many small vessels that arise from the pedicle.

In seventy cases we have seen three arteries with atypical courses. As the dissection proceeds, the flap is elevated from the tendon of the palmaris longus muscle, if present, and the tendon of the flexor carpi radialis muscle. Intermuscular septa that span the superficial fascia of the muscle bellies and their tendons must be cut through.

Several superficial veins must be ligated when removing the flap from the distal region. The dissection should not go too far distally, so as to avoid injury to the extensor retinaculum, which is anchored into the skin.

In the distal region, the pedicle that lies on the flexor pollicis longus muscle is directly lateral to the tendon of the flexor carpi radialis muscle. It is freed from the loose connective tissue layers between the vessels and muscle. Attention must be paid to large vessels that sometimes branch from the radial artery into the musculature. The pedicle is bound laterally by the tendon of

the brachioradialis muscle. The radial artery is sought in the distal edge of the flap and is cut and ligated together with the venae comitantes. It is advisable to fix sutures from the artery to the distal edge of the flap, so that it does not shear off during the procedure. Next the flap is dissected from the radial side.

The skin is dissected together with the fascia up to the abductor pollicis longus muscle and medially as far as the tendon of the brachioradialis muscle. The superficial branch of the radial nerve must be protected. To avoid a bad cosmetic result in the donor area, the dissection should not extend too far laterally. The pedicle is then dissected freed from the tendon of the brachioradialis muscle, during which it is important to pay attention to small branches. Next connective tissue septa that connect the pedicle with the radius, the intermuscular fascia, are cut through. Many small vessels will be found in this fascia that must either be coagulated or ligated.

Further dissection takes place along the pedicle (Fig. 2.**8**). At this point it must be decided whether to dissect the cephalic vein. This appears easy because it is bedded in a loose connective tissue sheath and has only a few veins feeding to it along a longer stretch proximal to the flap.

The pedicle is dissected from distal to proximal together with the fascia of the flexor digitorum superficialis muscle. Several vessels, some of them large, enter the muscle and must be ligated. Smaller vessels can be coagulated. The pedicle is dissected up to the proximal edge of the flap. First the radial artery and then the accompanying veins, or a deep vein into which they open, are ligated and cut.

For reconstruction of the mandible a forearm flap can be removed with a segment of radius up to 10 cm long. However, because significant cosmetic defects can arise in the donor area and spontaneous fracture may occur, we advise against using this osteocutaneous transplant.

However, if a section of the radius is included in the flap, the intermuscular septum that spans from the deep forearm fascia to the radius and contains the nourishing vessels must be preserved.

The dissection of the flap in a lateral direction is identical with that described above. Before the pedicle is reached from the ulnar side, the flexor pollicis longus, flexor digitorum superficialis, and pronator quadratus muscles are divided to the radius. This ensures that the musculoperiostal vessels running from the radial artery down

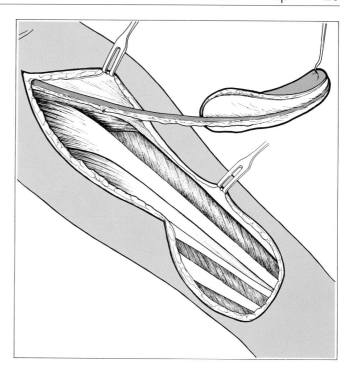

Fig. 2.**8**   After the flap has been lifted from its bed it is dissected together with the pedicle up to the proximal edge. The radial artery and its accompanying veins are removed together with the fascia of the flexor digitorum sublimis muscle.

to the bone remain intact. The segment of radius that spans the points of attachment of the pronator teres muscle and the brachioradialis muscle can be removed. In this way it is possible to obtain a piece of bone up to 10 cm long. On the lateral side the radius is exposed by lifting the brachioradialis muscle and the extensores carpi radialis brevis and longus muscles; then the radius can be split along its length with a saw.

Closure of the Donor Defect

Primary closure of the donor site is only possible with small distal flaps. The skin incision must lie far laterally to allow its medially based flap to be advanced distally.

We cover the defect with split skin from the thigh or the medial aspect of the upper arm (Fig. 2.9a). The graft is cut smaller than the defect, so that the resulting tension achieves a broad and flat coverage of the muscle and tendons. Wound healing over tendons is particularly difficult. Care should be taken not to injure the paratenon during flap dissection because otherwise the split skin will not heal and the tendon will become exposed. The dorsal surface of the forearm is splinted for 10 days, to immobilize the hand so that the split skin can heal undisturbed and does not shear off the tendons (Fig. 2.9b).

The most common complication at the donor site is flexor tendon exposure due either to injury

to the paratenon or inadequate immobilization. Then the split skin cannot heal over the tendon; usually, however, it is possible to cover the defect with a new split skin graft. It is also possible to injure the superficial branch of the radial nerve, which lies lateral to the radial artery and the tendon of the brachioradialis muscle, resulting in loss of sensation around the carpometacarpal joint of the thumb. If the donor site does not heal smoothly, scars and contractures may develop.

References

Chicarilli, Z. N., S. Ariyan, C. B. Cuono: Free radial forearm flap versatility for the head and neck and lower extremity. J. reconstr. Microsurg. 2 (1986) 221–228

Fatah, M. F., J. D. Nacarrow, D. S. Murray: Raising the radial artery forearm flap: the superficial ulnar artery "trap". Brit. J. plast. Surg. 38 (1985) 394–397

Lovie, M. J., G. M. Duncan, D. W. Glasson: Ulnar artery forearm free flap. Brit. J. plast. Surg. 37 (1984) 486

McGregor, A. D.: The free radial forearm flap – the management of the secondary defect. Brit. J. plast. Surg. 40 (1987) 83–85

Mühlbauer, W., E. Herndel, W. Stock: The forearm flap. Plast. reconstr. Surg. 70 (1982) 336–342

Soutar, D. S., L. R. Scheker, N. S. B. Tanner, I. A. McGregor: The radial forearm flap: a versatile method for intra-oral reconstruction. Brit. J. plast. Surg. 36 (1983) 1–8

Timmons, M. J.: The vascular basis of the radial forearm flap. Plast. reconstr. Surg. 77 (1986) 80–92

Yang, G., B. Chen, Y. Gao, X. Liu, J. Li, S. Jiang, S. He: Forearm free skin flap transplantation. Nat. med. J. China 61 (1981) 139

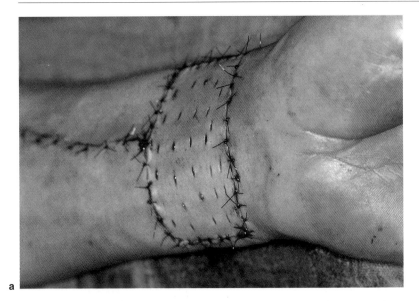

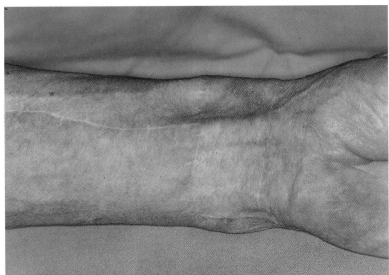

Fig. 2.**9** Closure of the donor site with split skin from the thigh. **a** The dermatome is set to a thickness of from 0.5 to 0.6 mm. In order to avoid hematoma the split skin is punctured with tiny slits. **b** Split skin that has taken and healed, 6 months after operation.

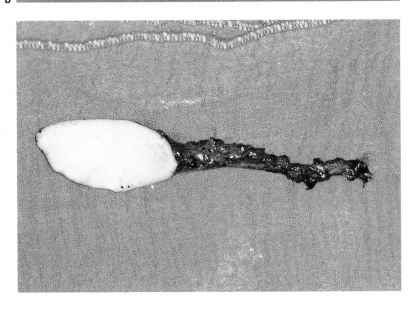

Fig. 2.**10** A small dorsalis pedis flap with the dorsalis pedis artery and its venae comitantes.

Dorsalis Pedis Flap

The dorsalis pedis flap (Fig. 2.10) is a fasciocutaneous graft, that, like the forearm flap, is well suited to reconstructing superficial defects in the head and neck. Unlike the forearm flap its size is limited to approximately 7 x 10 cm, so that larger defects cannot be covered with this flap. It is less commonly used now that the forearm flap has become increasingly popular, but is available when the latter is impractable or rejected by the patient. Because it has such a thin subcutaneous layer, this skin flap can be modeled very well and is particularly useful in reconstruction in the mouth and the pharynx. Almost the entire skin of the dorsum of the foot can be used as it is mainly supplied by the dorsalis pedis artery. The blood supply of the flap itself comes from the first dorsal metatarsal artery arising from the dorsalis pedis artery. The skin of the dorsum of the foot has a well-developed vascular supply. Either the usually paired venae comitantes of the dorsalis pedis artery and/or the cutaneous veins that drain into the great saphenous vein can be used for the venous anastomosis. We prefer the deep veins. The dorsalis pedis flap can be harvested as a small fasciocutaneous flap, or as a composite graft with muscle and bone, for example, a part of the second metatarsal bone. The possibility of removing the second toe with tendons and nerves for use in reconstruction of the hand is mentioned here only as an aside. It is not recommended because of the complication rate at the donor site.

Vascular Anatomy

The dorsalis pedis artery, which arises from the anterior tibial artery, is a robust vessel with a diameter of approximately 2–3 mm at the level of the upper ankle joint (Fig. 2.11). Small arteries branch off medially and laterally at the level of the upper ankle joint (anterior medial and lateral malleolar arteries). The dorsalis pedis artery is covered only by skin, subcutaneous tissue and fascia on the dorsum of the foot. After crossing under the tendon of the extensor hallucis brevis muscle it runs on the lateral side of the tendon of the extensor hallucis longus muscle (Fig. 2.12). The pulse can be felt in this area over the navicular or intermediate cuneiform bones. The arcuate artery is arch-shaped and runs laterally, is covered by the tendon of the extensor digitorum brevis muscle, and arises at the level of the tarsometatarsal joint. The dorsal metatarsal arteries

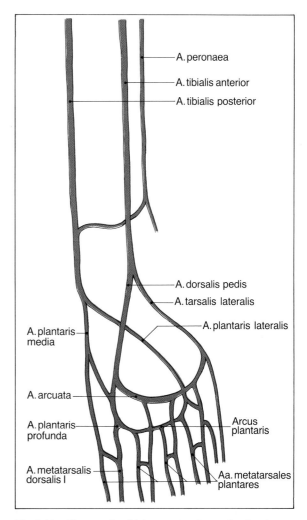

Fig. 2.11   The anterior tibial artery continues distal to the extensor retinaculum as the dorsalis pedis artery. The anterior medial and lateral malleolar arteries arise near the ankle joint. Further distally the lateral tarsal artery arises laterally and the medial tarsal arteries arise medially. The arcuate artery originates even further distally and runs over the base of the metatarsal bones to the side of the edge of the foot, where it anastomoses with the lateral tarsal artery. The dorsalis pedis artery breaks up into its end arteries, the first dorsal metatarsal and the deep plantar arteries, over the first metatarsal interosseous space.

arise from the arcuate, and run distally in the interosseal space over the second to fourth dorsal interossei muscles. The size of the flap determines whether the arcuate artery must be preserved.

The dorsalis pedis artery runs between the first and second metatarsal at the level of the first phalanx into the deep plantar artery, which then plunges towards the plantar aspect. The dorsalis pedis artery continues dorsally at this point as the first metatarsal artery, and runs on the first

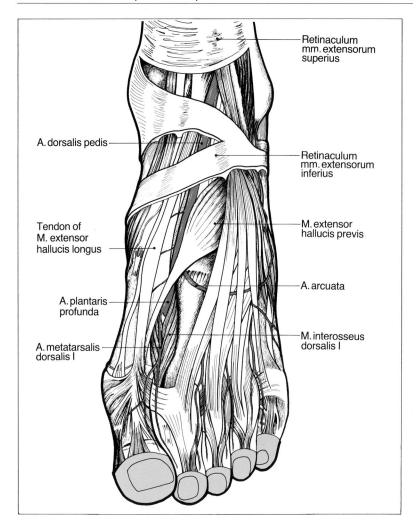

Retinaculum mm. extensorum superius

A. dorsalis pedis

Retinaculum mm. extensorum inferius

Tendon of M. extensor hallucis longus

M. extensor hallucis previs

A. arcuata

A. plantaris profunda

M. interosseus dorsalis I

A. metatarsalis dorsalis I

Fig. 2.**12**   The dorsalis pedis artery courses under the extensor retinaculum at the level of the ankle joint. Then it runs under the tendon of the extensor hallucis brevis muscle and divides distal to it into the first dorsal metatarsal artery and the deep plantar artery, that runs to the sole of the foot. The deep plantar artery runs between the heads of the first dorsal interosseus muscle and joins the lateral plantar artery to form the plantar arterial arch.

dorsal interosseus muscle to the great toe, dividing into two dorsal digital arteries. The first metatarsal artery lies 75% of the time either subcutaneously or buried in the upper layers of the first dorsal interosseus muscle (according to Gilbert). In these cases an adequate blood supply to the overlying skin is guaranteed. In 25% of cases the dorsal metatarsal artery runs through the lower layers of the interdigital muscle; then the blood supply is only adequate if the entire interosseus tissue is included in the dissection. Small vessels running to the skin arise in the proximal and distal area of the dorsal metatarsal artery. These can always be exposed distally between the great and second toe, lying beneath the skin in the interdigital space, so that elevating the flap retrograde from this point is easy. The arterial network on the dorsum of the foot varies greatly, as described above, and it must be considered during the removal of the flap. This is particu-

larly true of the arcuate and dorsal metatarsal arteries.

The most well-perfused region of the fasciocutaneous flap is over the first and second metatarsal bones. The longer the pedicle needed, the further distal the flap should lie.

The flap is drained adequately by the deep venous system of the venae comitantes that accompany the dorsalis pedis artery. The great saphenous vein, which collects the blood from the epifascial veins lying in the loose subcutaneous tissue of the dorsum of the foot, can also be dissected. It runs on the medial edge of the foot in front of the medial ankle. The deep peroneal nerve stretches medial to the dorsalis pedis artery over the dorsum of the foot and continues with its end branches in the first interosseal space, where it divides into the dorsal digital pedis nerves and supplies the skin in the space between the first and second toes.

Flap Planning

The status of the vessels in the leg to be operated on must be ascertained in the preoperative planning. Disease of the arteries or intermittent claudication contraindicate this flap. It must also be ensured that the posterior tibial artery or the peroneal artery can provide sufficient perfusion for the foot when the dorsalis pedis artery is divided. A palpable posterior tibial and dorsalis pedis pulse is not proof that both vessels have forward flow, because the vessels can have retrograde flow if a stenosis lies higher up or a blockage in the lower leg is present. There must be a palpable pulse over the dorsalis pedis artery when the posterior tibial artery is occluded and there must be a pulse over the posterior tibial artery when the dorsalis pedis artery is occluded. Only when the pulse is still palpable in one vessel while the other is compressed can it be assumed that both vessels are open to orthograde perfusion.

The course of the dorsalis pedis artery is palpated and is drawn on the skin (Fig. 2.**13**); the proximal veins of the skin, i.e., the vessels feeding the great saphenous vein, are marked as well. Because the flap is very thin, the size can be estimated exactly allowing for a 20% retraction in size. Dissection is best carried out from lateral to medial and from distal to proximal. The outline of the flap is drawn on the dorsum of the foot (Fig. 2.**13**) so that the axis lies over the second metatarsal bone.

Flap Elevation

The flap is incised around its edges marked on the skin; the dissection begins laterally and moves medially (Figs. 2.**14**, 2.**15**). The incision reaches the paratenon of the extensor tendon, which must be protected. The flap is lifted up to the tendon of the extensor digitorum longus muscle of the second toe. Then it is dissected from the distal edge; the first dorsal metatarsal artery, which lies superficially on the distal edge of the flap on the interosseal musculature, is identified and divided (Fig. 2.**16**). The distal end is sutured to the subcutaneous tissue to prevent the artery from separating from the flap and endangering the perfusion. If the first dorsal metatarsal artery runs inside the first dorsal interosseus muscle, the muscle is removed with the flap. The flap must now be lifted from the medial edge towards the tendon of the extensor hallucis longus muscle (Fig. 2.**17**).

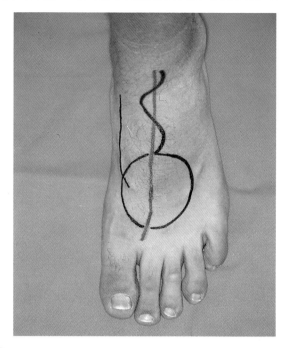

Fig. 2.**13** Before the flap is removed its outline is marked on the dorsum of the foot, along with the course of the dorsalis pedis artery and the great saphenous vein.

The dissection continues along the first dorsal metatarsal artery as far as the origin of the deep plantar artery from the dorsalis pedis artery. When the deep plantar artery, needed for plantar arterial blood supply, has been identified, the rest of the pedicle that serves to guide the dissection of the flap into the first and second interdigital space can easily be developed proximally. The venae comitantes that run parallel are vulnerable and should not be injured. Tributaries should be ligated so that the ligatures do not narrow the vena comitans. The use of vascular clips can speed up the procedure considerably. The tendon of the extensor hallucis brevis muscle, stretching over the dorsalis pedis artery proximal to the origin of the deep plantar artery must always be divided in the dissection of the flap. This step has no sequelae, because the tendon has no essential function. The pedicle can then be followed further proximally. At the level of the ankle joint the retinacula of the extensor tendons are divided, but they must be sutured together after the flap has been removed in order to close the defect.

If a very long pedicle is required, an S-shaped skin incision on the ventral side of the distal lower leg is used. A dorsalis pedis flap with sensory innervation is provided by including a superficial branch of the peroneus nerve that

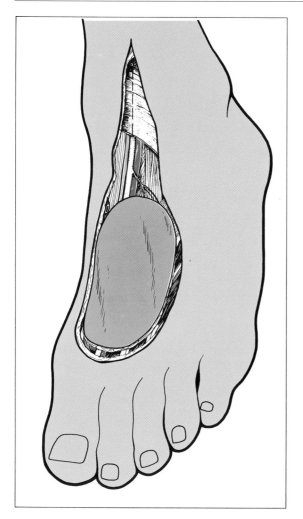

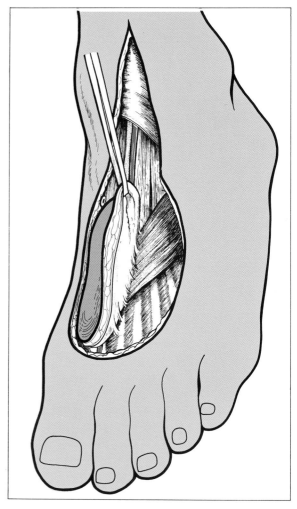

Fig. 2.14   The flap is first incised along its superior edges distal to the extensor retinaculum, which will be divided later in the dissection (dashed line). The first metatarsal artery is exposed in the interdigital cleft in the subcutaneous tissue between the great toe and the second toe in the distal part of the flap.

Fig. 2.15   The dissection of the flap is carried out from lateral to medial, the incision being carried down to the paratenon of the extensor tendons. The flap is elevated from the tendon of the extensor digitorum longus muscle of the second toe. The flap is turned back and dissected further in a proximal direction.

courses from lateral to medial at the level of the lateral malleolus over the superficial fascia to supply the skin of the dorsum of the foot up to the proximal part of the toes. The deep branch of the peroneus nerve runs together with the dorsalis pedis artery and supplies the skin of the first interdigital space.

Closure of the Donor Defect

The paratenon must be protected carefully while lifting the flap, to preserve the extensor tendon and to ensure that the split skin heals (Fig. 2.18).

We use carefully fitted split skin 0.4–0.6 mm thick to close the donor site under a bolus dress-

ing to ensure good contact between the graft and its bed because the space between the first and second metatarsal is particularly deep after the flap has been removed. Careful hemostasis is important to avoid a subcutaneous hematoma. Tourniquets are not used while elevating the flap, so that hemostasis can be performed during the dissection.

The great disadvantage of the dorsalis pedis flap is the donor defect, which demands immobilization of the patient that can lead to a difficult convalescence, particularly with high-risk patients because of compromise of lung function, and the risk of thrombosis. The donor limb cannot bear weight for 14 days; we order abso-

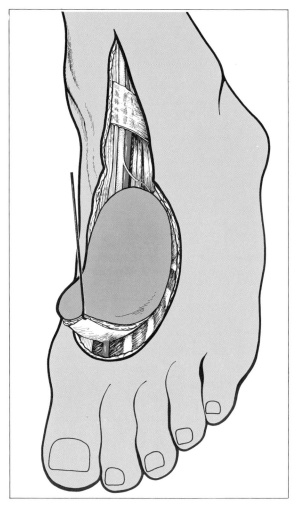

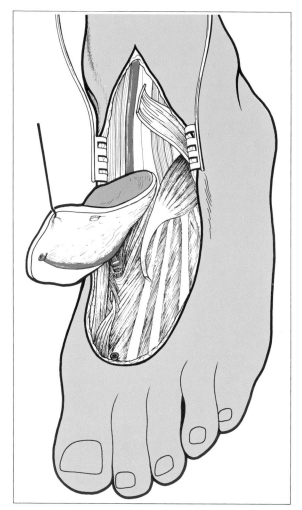

Fig. 2.**16**   The first dorsal metatarsal artery is identified at the distal edge of the flap, lying on the interosseous musculature, and divided. If it runs within the first dorsal interosseous muscle, the muscle is included in the flap.

Fig. 2.**17**   The further dissection is carried out from the medial side down to the tendon of the extensor hallucis longus muscle, then along the first dorsal metatarsal artery to the point where the deep plantar artery leaves the dorsalis pedis. After the deep plantar artery is ligated and the tendon of the extensor hallucis brevis has been divided, the pedicle can be easily dissected in a proximal direction. Because the pedicle runs proximally under the extensor retinaculum, the latter must be divided.

lute bed rest for 5 days until the bolus dressing can be removed. If the skin has healed with no signs of inflammation, we start the first passive movement excercises in bed. After 14 days the patient can be fully mobilized.

References

Gilbert, A.: Composite tissue transfers from the foot: anatomic basis and surgical technique. In Daniller, A., B. Strauch: Symposium on Microsurgery, Vol. 15. Mosby, St. Louis 1976

Huber, J. F.: The arterial network supplying the dorsum of the foot. Anat. Rec. 80 (1941) 343

Man, D., R. D. Acland: The microarterial anatomy of the dorsalis pedis flap and its clinical application. Plast. reconstr. Surg. 65 (1980) 419

McCraw, J. B., L. T. Furlow jr.: The dorsalis pedis arterialized flap. A clinical study. Plast. reconstr. Surg. 55 (1975) 177

Morrison, W. A., B. McC. O'Brien, A. M. MacLeod: The foot as a donor site in reconstructive microsurgery. Wld J. Surg. 3 (1979) 43–52

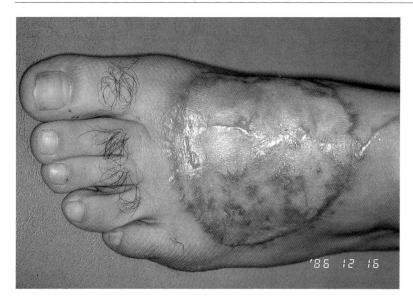

Fig. 2.**18**   Closure of the donor site with split skin graft. Appearance 3 months later.

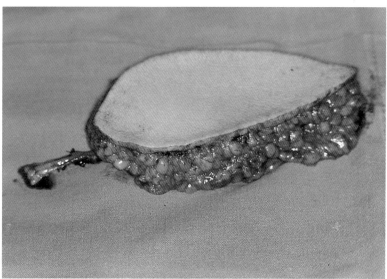

Fig. 2.**19**   Scapluar flap with a short pedicle that was elevated using a simple dissection between the teres major and the teres minor muscles.

Scapular and Parascapular Flaps

The scapular flap (Fig. 2.**19**) was first described by Dos Santos in 1980. The cutaneous graft is popular because of its reliable vascular pedicle. The circumflex scapular artery with its accompanying veins has a large diameter and offers ideal qualities for microvascular anastomosis. The pedicle can be as long as 10 cm if the subscapular artery is included. The thickness of the flap is extremely variable, but it is usually thinner than the groin flap. The scapular flap can be used for augmentation in the facial region as well as for reconstruction after removal of larger external tumors of the head and neck. Together with a bone segment it can be used for reconstruction of the mandible. In almost all cases it is possible to close the donor defect primarily but the scars spread due to the tension on the suture, so that the cosmetic result is often not completely satisfying, particularly for women.

Vascular Anatomy

The subscapular artery arises from the axillary artery, divides into the thoracodorsal and the circumflex scapular arteries (Fig. 2.**20**). The circumflex scapular artery courses through the space between the teres major and minor muscles to reach the skin over the scapula (Fig. 2.**21**).

It runs on the lateral edge of the scapula and gives off branches to the bone. The circumflex scapular artery divides into two branches, one running horizontally and one vertical. The two vessels nourish the scapular and parascapular flaps. The subscapular artery has a diameter of about 3 to 4 mm, the circumflex scapular artery from 2 to 3 mm or more.

Flap Planning

The flap is removed while the patient is lying on his side with the arm abducted.

First the anatomical landmarks are drawn on the skin (Figs. 2.22, 2.23), namely the spine of the scapula, the inferior angle, and the lateral edge of the scapula. The space between the teres minor and major muscles, which can be felt on the lateral edge of the scapula, is also marked. The pedicle emerges through this opening between the muscle that is limited superiorly by the long head of the triceps muscle, that is the point through which the axes of the scapular and parascapular flaps run. The axis of the scapular flap is parallel to the spine of the scapula, whereas the axis of the parascapular flap is parallel to the lateral edge of the scapula. The shape of the flap should be chosen so that the ends meet at a sharp angle, in order that the donor defect can be primarily closed.

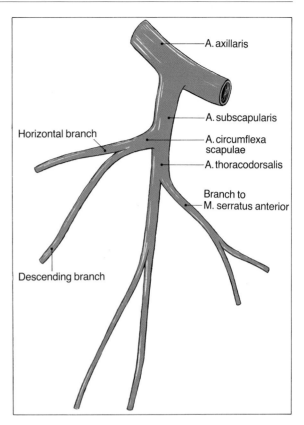

Fig. 2.**20**   The circumflex scapular artery, which supplies the scapular or parascapular flap, leaves the subscapular artery about 2 to 4 cm distal to the axillary artery.

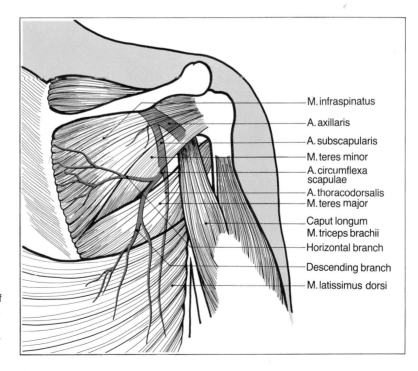

Fig. 2.**21**   The circumflex scapular artery runs through the intramuscular space between the teres major and minor muscles over the lateral edge of the scapula into the subcutaneous tissue of the skin over the scapula. Shortly thereafter it divides into a horizontal and a descending branch.

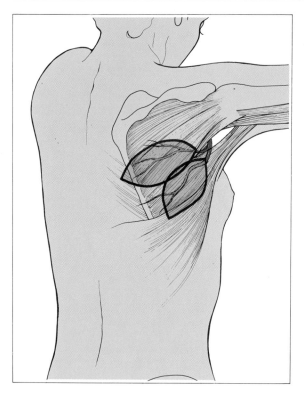

Fig. 2.**22** The flap can be elevated as a scapular flap with a skin island, with an axis parallel to the spine of the scapula and blood supply from the horizontal branch of the circumflex scapular artery. The axis of the parascapular flap runs parallel to the lateral edge of the scapula and is carried by the descending branch of the circumflex scapular artery.

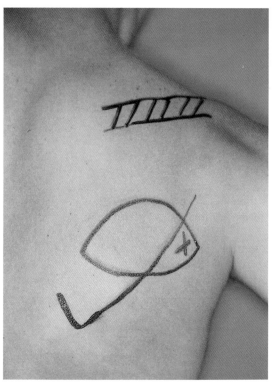

Fig. 2.**23** The anatomical landmarks, such as the spine of the scapula, the inferior angle, and the lateral edge of the scapula are drawn on the skin while planning the flap. The point where the pedicle is to be found in the space between the teres minor and major muscles is also marked.

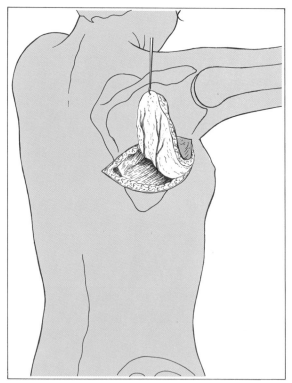

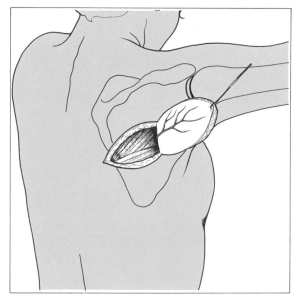

Fig. 2.**25** The flap is dissected further in an inferolateral direction until the pedicle is reached.

◀ Fig. 2.**24** The dissection of the flap begins medially with an incision extending to the fascia of the infraspinatus muscle.

Flap Elevation

The dissection of the flap begins medially; the incision reaches to the fascia of the infraspinatus muscle, which should be left intact (Fig. 2.24). The dissection is carried out from lateroinferior towards the pedicle, which can be recognized by the small vessel branches to the skin (Fig. 2.25). Next the vessels between the teres minor and major muscles are exposed and separated by retractors to dissect an appropriate length of pedicle (Fig. 2.26). The flap can now be completely incised around its edges. There are several vessel branches to ligate that enter the musculature and the scapula. Using this procedure, a pedicle of 6–8 cm in length can be dissected. However, it is not possible to lengthen the pedicle by inclusion of the subscapular artery using this access. If this is required, an access over the axilla must be developed through which the circumflex scapular artery with the subscapular artery extending up to the axillary artery can be removed.

If it is seen during flap elevation that a longer pedicle is needed, the first step in the dissection can be carried out through the axilla, in which the subscapular artery and its continuation in the thoracodorsal artery are exposed (see Fig. 2.20). The first large vessel branching dorsally, the circumflex scapular artery, is followed from medial to dorsal, under and through the point of attachment of the latissimus dorsi muscle near the humerus. First the flap is incised at this point as described above. When the flap is fully dissected it can be pulled through the space between the teres major and minor muscles towards the axilla. After smaller vessels and the thoracodorsal artery have been ligated, the pedicle is dissected as far as the axillary artery and divided, providing a pedicle with a length of up to 10 cm.

The scapular flap can be elevated with a bone segment from the scapula (Fig. 2.27). This is taken either from the lateral edge or the spine of the scapula; we prefer the former (Fig. 2.28). During the dissection, carried out as described up to the point where the pedicle emerges in the intramuscular space between the teres minor and major muscles, attention must be paid to the small vessels leaving the circumflex scapular artery at the lateral edge and coursing into the bone. The length of the bone segment is marked on the lateral edge of the scapula or determined by the use of a template. The infraspinatus muscle is incised down to the periosteum about 3–4 cm medial to the lateral edge of the scapula, and elevated from the scapula in the area of

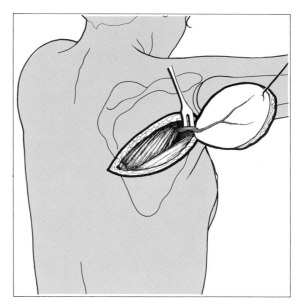

Fig. 2.**26**   The pedicle is followed in the space between the teres major and minor muscles after separating the two muscles from each other. Several branches run to the lateral edge of the scapula: if a cutaneous flap is needed these vessels can be divided but if a bony segment is to be removed, they must be preserved.

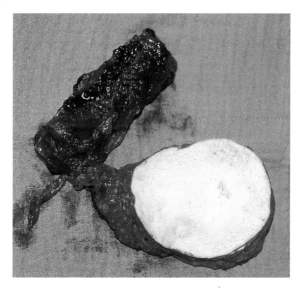

Fig. 2.**27**   Osteocutaneous scapular flap, harvested using a combined access via the axilla, allowing the pedicle to be dissected up to the axillary artery and vein.

the planned bone incision with a raspatory (Fig. 2.29).

Because the infraspinatus muscle usually fuses with the teres minor muscle in its lower part, they must be separated from each other. To avoid endangering the vessel as it enters the bone, a 1–2 cm broad stretch of teres minor mus-

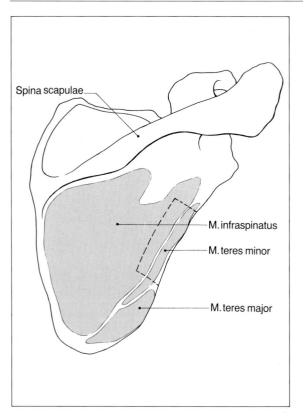

Fig. 2.**28**   The lateral edge of the scapula is particularly well suited as a donor site for a segment of bone.

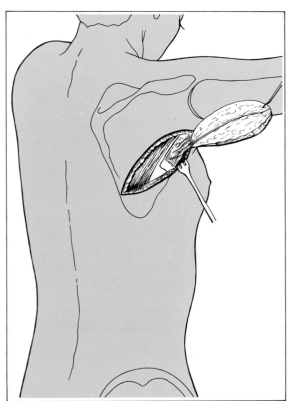

cle is left on the lateral edge of the scapula. The segment of bone is removed with an oscillating saw, respecting the glenoid lip above, to prevent injury to the shoulder joint. The bone segment is carefully lifted from above downwards and separated from the underlying subscapular muscle, preserving a small strip of muscle.

The defect is closed primarily by undermining the surrounding skin.

References

Baker, S. R., M. J. Sullivan: Osteocutaneous free scapular flap for one stage mandibular reconstruction. Arch. Otolaryngol. 114 (1988) 267–277

Barwick, W. J., D. J. Goodkind, B. Serafin: The free scapular flap. Plast. reconstr. Surg. 69 (1982) 779

Dos Santos, L. F.: The vascular anatomy and dissection of the free scapular flap. Plast. reconstr. Surg. 73 (1982) 59

Gilbert, A., L. Teot: The free scapular flap. Plast. reconstr. Surg. 69 (1982) 601

Mayou, B. J., D. Whitby, B. M. Jones: The scapular flap – an anatomical and clinical study. Brit. J. plast. Surg. 35 (1982) 8

Nassif, T. M., L. Vidal, J. L. Povet, J. Baudet: The parascapular flap: a new cutaneous microsurgical free flap. Plast. reconstr. Surg. 69 (1982) 591–600

Urbaniak, J. R., L. A. Koman, R. D. Goldner, N. B. Armstrong, J. A. Nunley: The vascularized cutaneous scapular flap. Plast. reconstr. Surg. 69 (1982) 772–778

Latissimus Dorsi Flap

The most commonly used musculocutaneous flap is the latissimus dorsi flap (Fig. 2.**30**). It is part of the standard repertoire in reconstructive surgery—its size and versatility make it an extraordinary graft. It can be used for covering defects in every part of the body, because it is a composite graft in which variable amounts of muscle, skin, and subcutaneous tissue can be included. It can be as large as 20 x 25 x 40 cm. The skin is nourished via the fascia, which therefore must be removed with the muscle. It is possible to use the muscle alone as a free graft (Fig. 2.**31**). The latissimus dorsi flap can be elevated with the serratus muscle and the accompanying rib or with a scap-

◀ Fig. 2.**29**   To remove a segment of bone from the scapula, the infraspinatus muscle must be pushed medially away from the bone. To preserve the bone's vascular supply, a strip of muscle must be left on the lateral edge of the scapula, consisting of parts of the teres major and minor muscles. Once the bony segment is freely exposed it is removed with an oscillating saw. The subscapular muscle, which inserts on the posterior surface of the scapula at this point, is divided.

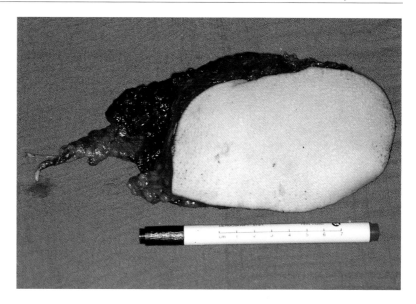

Fig. 2.**30** Latissimus dorsi flap with subscapular artery and vein.

ular or parascapular flap on the same pedicle. In this way it is possible to cover complex defects simultaneously with several flaps. The muscle adducts and rotates the arm medially at the shoulder joint; loss of this function does not usually disturb the patient. For a patient who has a transverse lesion of the spinal cord with paraplegia however, the resulting limitation in movement makes the muscle functionally very important. In this case, the latissimus dorsi flap must not be used.

Vascular Anatomy

The vascular bundle that nourishes the muscle originates in the axillary artery and vein. It courses as the subscapular artery and vein in the middle of the axilla parallel and inferior to the edge of the latissimus dorsi muscle (Fig. 2.**32**). About 2–4 cm distal to the axillary artery the circumflex scapular artery and vein arise from the subscapular artery and course as the thoracodorsal artery and vein to the latissimus dorsi muscle, which it penetrates about 10–12 cm from the axillary artery (Fig. 2.**33**). Shortly before it enters the muscle, the vascular bundle gives off an arciform artery to the serratus anterior muscle. The latissimus dorsi muscle is nourished by at least two arciform arteries: one parallel to the anterior edge, lying about 1–2 cm from the edge, and another main arcade that courses at an angle to supply the dorsal and medial part of the muscle. From this last arcade arise many smaller arcades, which extend from the origin to the insertion of the muscle. Towards the inferior end of the muscle insertion are to be found several vascular arcades that are connected to the serratus anterior muscle and must be divided when the flap is elevated.

Because only relatively small flaps are needed for reconstruction in the head and neck, the flap can be elevated with the patient lying on his back. The flap should be raised directly over the ventral edge of the muscle, because about 1.2 cm dorsal to it lies a main vessel arcade, which gives off small perforating vessels running through the muscle to the skin. The caliber of the vessels that nourish the flap varies according to which pedicle is used. If dissection is continued up to the ax-

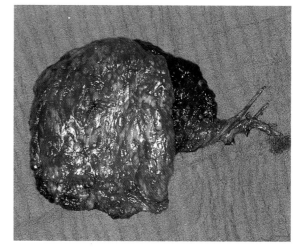

Fig. 2.**31**   Latissimus dorsi flap consisting of muscle only.

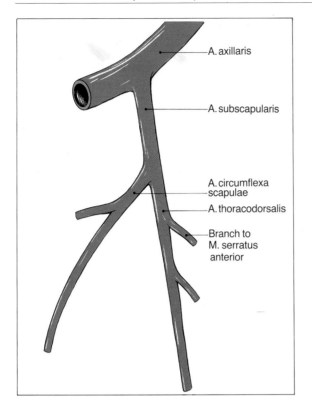

Fig. 2.**32**   The thoracodorsal artery, which supplies the latissimus dorsi muscle, is a direct extension of the subscapular artery. Shortly before the origin of the circumflex scapular artery, another vascular bundle arises and runs forwards to the serratus anterior muscle.

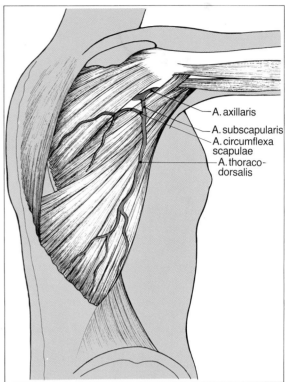

Fig. 2.**33**   The thoracodorsal artery runs parallel to and about 2 cm posterior to the anterior edge of the latissimus dorsi muscle, which it enters about 10–12 cm distal to the axillary artery.

illary artery, the artery can have a diameter of up to 4 mm. The diameter is on an average 2.5 mm distal to the origin of the circumflex scapular artery, and the thoracodorsal artery as it enters the muscle is usually less than 2 mm thick. The veins are often present in pairs up to the branching of the circumflex scapular artery, but then they often unite to form a single vein that courses to the axilla. This can be up to 4 mm in diameter. The pedicle can be as long as 14 cm.

The thoracodorsal nerve accompanies the pedicle; it must be divided, but there is no loss of function.

Flap Planning

The proportion of skin to muscle must be exactly determined during preoperative planning. The flap can be varied according to the requirements for skin or muscle. If more skin than muscle is needed, then the skin island should be based upon the anterior edge of the muscle. This extends far anteriorly by as much as 10 cm with the

muscle being about 5 cm broad (Fig. 2.**34**). Several areas of skin can be lifted separately on the same muscle flap, so that many reconstruction possibilities are available. The anterior edge of the muscle should always be included because the greatest number of perforating vessels supplying the skin are found there. Before the operation it is easy to find the anterior edge of the muscle. It can be seen and felt when the hands are placed on the hips.

First a line is drawn from the middle of the iliac crest to the posterior axillary fold. The entry of the pedicle into the musculature 12 cm below the axilla is marked on the line. After the size of the skin flap has been determined, it is drawn on the skin with the help of a template, so that the line described above lies on the axis of the flap to be elevated (Fig. 2.**35**).

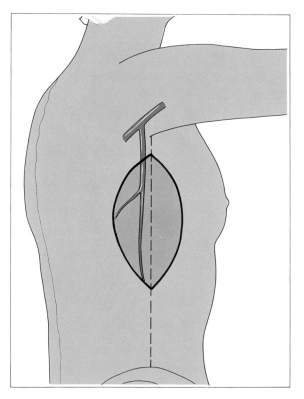

Fig. 2.**34**   The axis of the flap lies about 2 cm posterior to the anterior edge of the latissimus dorsi muscle; the skin island can be anterior to this edge of the muscle. Ideally the flap is based on the anterior edge of the muscle because there is a concentration of perforating vessels in this area.

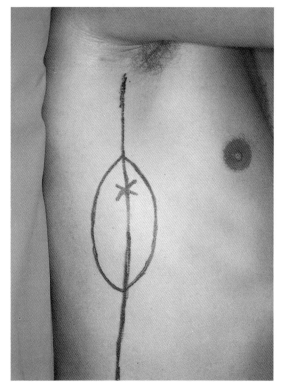

Fig. 2.**35**   When planning the flap, a line is drawn from the posterior axillary fold to the middle of the iliac spine, and the entry of the pedicle about 10–12 cm distal to the axilla is marked.

Flap Elevation

We always orient ourselves on the anterior edge of the latissimus dorsi muscle, in an area extending from the axilla to the point of entry of the pedicle into the musculature. From this point it is easy to expose the border between the muscle and the connective tissue on the anterior edge of the latissimus dorsi with a skin incision in the direction of the axilla and the chest wall (Fig. 2.**36**). The course of the pedicle is relatively constant, about 1–2 cm behind the anterior edge of the muscle. The dissection is carried out about a hand's breadth under the axilla medial to the anterior edge of the latissimus. The arteriovenous vascular bundle lies in the fatty connective tissue between the medial surface of the muscle and the chest wall. The length of the pedicle is dissected towards the axilla and branches to the axillary artery and vein are exposed. These are ligated at the pedicle end with 4–0 sutures, clipped distally with vascular clamps, and then divided.

After the pedicle has been identified, the distal dissection is simple; the entry of the pedicle into the muscle is now exposed. The skin island is incised on its circumference and the latissimus dorsi muscle is lifted from the serratus anterior muscle by blunt dissection (Fig. 2.**37**). Distally the vessel arcades that run to the chest wall must be coagulated by diathermy. To prevent the skin from shearing off the muscle, it is sutured to it; if the skin extends beyond the muscle, its edge is adapted to the subcutis. Hemostasis must be performed immediately, because the vessels can retract, making later control more difficult. The incision of the muscle by diathermy results in less bleeding than when a scalpel or scissors are used, but it causes considerable muscle contraction, which can pull the flap out of shape. Therefore we prefer to cut the muscle with large scissors. We cut the inferior edge of the flap first obliquely and then posteriorly in the direction of the muscle fibers from below upwards. The anterior edge of the muscle must not be incised, so as to protect the blood supply. Larger vessels must be immediately ligated with absorbable 3–0 or 4–0

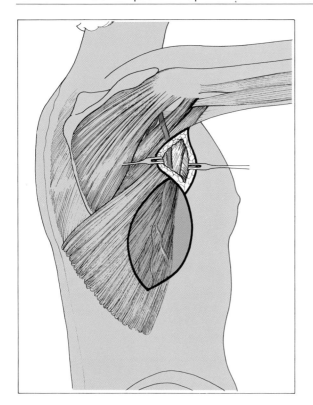

Fig. 2.**36**   The first preparatory incision exposes the anterior edge of the latissimus dorsi muscle between the axilla and the proximal edge of the flap. Then the pedicle is easily found in the fatty connective tissue medial to the muscle and exposed up to its entry into the latissimus dorsi muscle.

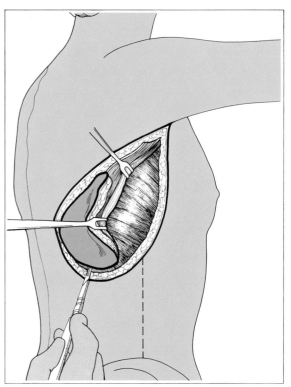

Fig. 2.**37**   Once the pedicle is exposed, the skin island is incised around its circumfrence and elevated anteriorly from the serratus anterior muscle up to the ventral edge of the latissimus dorsi muscle. Next the latissimus dorsi muscle with its overlying skin island is dissected bluntly from the serratus anterior muscle; sometimes sharp dissection is necessary caudally.

sutures, and smaller vessels can be coagulated. The muscle must be divided very carefully proximal to the entry of the thoracodorsal artery, so as to avoid injury to the pedicle (Fig. 2.**38**).

In this area the vessel arcade usually runs to the dorsal part of the latissimus dorsi muscle, which can be divided after ligature. In order to recognize possible bleeding, we leave the pedicle intact until the skin and the muscle are fully dissected and elevated. A careful hemostasis near the edges of the flap and on the back of the muscle to prevent later bleeding is better performed after the flap has been turned over. Control of bleeding in situ, particularly when the elevation is carried out in the prone position, is not always easy. The pedicle is divided later.

Closure of the Donor Defect

Before closing the donor site we insert two suction drains (size 14), one for the axilla and one for the lateral chest wall. The site is closed using strong absorbable subcutaneous sutures (for example, Dexon 0–0). The surrounding skin is undermined beforehand; this can be difficult with the patient in the prone position. A second continuous suture or a row of clips closes the skin and the pedicle is rinsed with a heparin–NaCl solution (5000 units/100 ml). The flap is protected between two wet swabs. A latissimus dorsi flap can be kept for several hours without danger of tissue damage.

The donor site can usually be closed primarily even with a flap up to 15 cm wide. This is easier to do when the patient is lying on his side. However, a primary closure should not be done under tension—a mesh graft can be used to cover the defect if necessary.

If the flap has a large skin island, the defect should be closed by a mesh graft. It is difficult to achieve aesthetic closure of these donor sites, particularly in obese patients. In these cases the edges of the defect can be thinned and adapted on the muscle bed using sutures or skin clips.

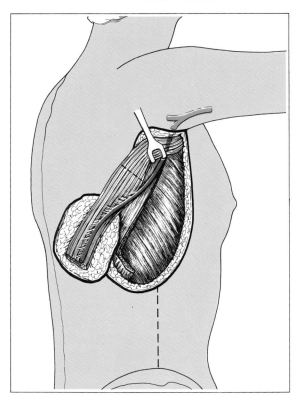

Fig. 2.**38** The latissimus dorsi muscle is divided below and posteriorly but remains still attached above. In this area (dashed line) the relatively small muscle is dissected free, protecting the pedicle carefully; a vessel branch running posteriorly must be ligated.

The mesh graft can then be more successfully applied and it heals better on the muscle bed. A mesh graft of 2.1 or 3:1 is typically used.

The suction drains are removed after 2–3 days, or when they accumulate less than 15 ml fluid in 24 hours. The skin clips or sutures are left for at least 20 days because of the tension. If the skin has been continuously sutured, the sutures should not be removed before 2 weeks. Mesh grafts are dressed until the fifth day after operation, and thereafter the dressings changed every second day. After 10 days the wound can usually be left without dressings.

We use physiotherapy only for older patients. If the donor region has been closed under great tension we start careful excercises of the affected shoulder on the fourth day, because limitation in movement quickly sets in owing to protective posturing.

References

Bartlett, S. P., J. W. May jr., J. M. Yaremchuk: The latissimus dorsi muscle. A fresh cadaver study of the primary neurovascular pedicle. Plast. reconstr. Surg. 67 (1981) 631–636

Barton jr., F. E., T. E. Spicer, H. S. Byrd: Head and neck reconstruction with the latissimus dorsi myocutaneous flap: Anatomic observations and report of 60 cases. Plast. reconstr. Surg. 71 (1983) 199–204

Maxwell, C. P., K. Stueber, J. Hoopes: A free latissimus dorsi myocutaneous flap. Plast. reconstr. Surg. 62 (1978) 462

Olivari, N.: The latissimus flap. Brit. J. plast. Surg. 29 (1976) 126

Quillen, G. C.: Latissimus dorsi myocutaneous flaps in head and neck reconstruction. Plast. reconstr. Surg. 63 (1979) 664–670

Watson, J. S., R. D. P. Craig, C. I. Orton: The free latissimus dorsi myocutaneous flap. Plast. reconstr. Surg. 64 (1979) 299

Rectus Abdominis Flap

The rectus abdominis muscle arises from the edge of the ribs, the xiphoid process, and the costoxiphoid ligaments and inserts into the upper edge of the pubic bone between the pubic tubercle and the symphysis. The muscle usually has three tendinous intersections at the level of the xiphoid, between the xiphoid and umbilicus, and at the level of the umbilicus. The tendinous insertions are firmly bound to the anterior layer of the rectus sheath, formed by the aponeuroses of the three lateral abdominal muscles. Beneath the arcuate line the three aponeuroses run in front of the rectus abdominis muscle. The posterior layer is absent in this area. Above the line, the anterior rectus sheath is composed of the aponeurosis of the external oblique muscle and the anterior half of the aponeurosis of the internal oblique muscle. The posterior layer is formed from the aponeurosis of the transverse muscle and the posterior half of the internal oblique muscle. The rectus sheath encases the rectus abdominis muscle.

The paired rectus abdominis muscles are supplied above and below by two vessel branches, from the inferior epigastric artery and vein and the superior epigastric artery and vein (Fig. 2.**39**). The muscle can use both vessels as a pedicle. The superior epigastric artery is always smaller than the inferior epigastric artery. There is more risk of venous insufficiency when the upper vessel arcade is used, than with the lower. The skin over the rectus muscle is nourished through the fascia by perforating vessels, much like the latissimus dorsi flap. The skin paddle

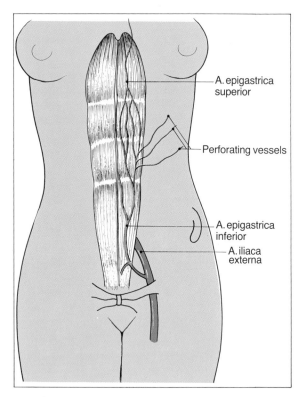

A. epigastrica superior

Perforating vessels

A. epigastrica inferior

A. iliaca externa

Fig. 2.**39**   The paired rectus abdominis muscle is supplied by two vessels, one from cranial, the other from caudal; that is, from the inferior and superior epigastric arteries. The inferior epigastric artery arises from the iliac artery, whereas the superior epigastric artery is a direct continuation of the internal thoracic artery. The branches of the inferior and superior epigastric arteries anastomose within the rectus abdominis muscle.

should not be much broader than the rectus muscle itself, otherwise problems may arise in closing the abdominal defect.

If more subcutaneous fat and skin tissue are needed, the skin can be lifted in an oblique oval shape from the lower third. It is thus possible to elevate a very large epigastric skin and muscle flap from the rectus abdominis (Fig. 2.**40**). The rectus muscle has the advantage that it can be removed while the patient is in the prone position.

Removal of the rectus muscle weakens the musculature of the abdominal wall considerably. Because there is sometimes a large amount of epigastric fatty tissue, the use of the rectus muscle is often limited because it is too bulky for constructive purposes.

The rectus muscle can be used as an isolated muscle graft, but it is not often used as a free transplant. Its advantages lie in its size, the ease of its harvesting, and the reliability of its pedicle.

The posterior rectus sheath can be removed with the muscle and the peritoneum. Such a graft of peritoneum, fascia, muscle, skin, and subcutaneous tissue can be used to cover multilayer defects, for example, in the cheek, where the peritoneum can be used to line the oral cavity.

Because of the disadvantages mentioned above, the rectus abdominis flap is the second choice after the latissimus dorsi flap for reconstruction in the head and neck.

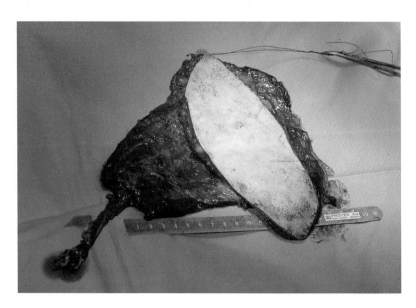

Fig. 2.**40**   Rectus abdominis flap based on the inferior epigastric vessels.

Vascular Anatomy

The inferior epigastric artery (Fig. 2.**41**) has a reliable course. It arises medially from the external iliac artery, proximal to the origin of the deep iliac circumflex artery. Rarely the inferior epigastric artery can arise from the femoral artery, just below the inguinal ligament. It has a diameter of 1.5–2.5 mm and is accompanied by one or two venae comitantes. These veins can be up to 4 mm thick and they drain into the external iliac vein.

The inferior epigastric artery enters the lower third of the rectus abdominis muscle laterally at the level of the arcuate line, where no posterior rectus sheath is present. The pedicle emerges from the extraperitoneal subfascial fatty tissue and runs along the lateral edge of the rectus abdominis muscle 6–7 cm above the symphysis. From this point the arteries run below or within the muscle itself towards the superior epigastric vessels, with which they anastomose. Usually the vessel gives off two or three branches as it runs superiorly. If fibers of the external oblique muscle are divided lengthwise in this region, the vessels are found external to the rectus sheath above the iliac vessels. The pampiniform plexus lies in this area in men. The superior epigastric artery and vein, which arise from the internal thoracic artery and vein, are less reliable than the lower epigastric vessels. The superior epigastric arteries are smaller than the inferior, being at most 2 mm thick. The veins are not much larger.

The main blood supply to the abdominal skin comes from the perforating branches of the epigastric vessels concentrated in the paraumbilical region (Fig. 2.**42**). The larger paraumbilical muscular perforating vessels run at an angle of 45°. For this reason skin flaps that run at an oblique angle have been developed, which sometimes extend far beyond the musculature.

Flap Planning

The position of the xiphoid process, the inferior border of the ribs, the pubic bone, and the position of the rectus abdominis muscle are marked on the skin (Fig. 2.**43**). The entry of the inferior epigastric artery is marked approximately in the middle between the umbilicus and the pubic bone on the lateral border of the rectus abdominis muscle. The flap is drawn on the skin lengthwise for small flaps, or at an oblique lateral an-

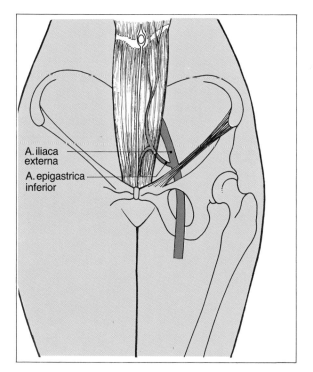

Fig. 2.**41**   The inferior epigastric artery arises directly behind the inguinal ligament, to enter the lower third of the rectus abdominis muscle laterally at the level of the arcuate line, 6–7 cm above the symphysis.

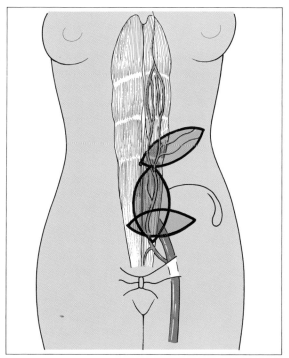

Fig. 2.**42**   The perforator vessels, which are particularly concentrated in the paraumbilical region, run at an angle of 45°, so that oblique cutaneous flaps can be elevated, extending partly beyond the muscle. Proximal to this, flaps can be elevated either parallel or perpendicular to the rectus abdominis muscle.

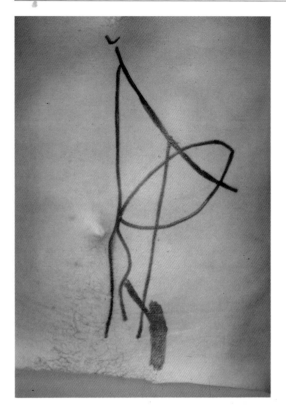

Fig. 2.**43**   The xiphoid process, the lower edge of the ribs, and the pubic bone are drawn on the skin, and the position of the rectus abdominis muscle is marked.

gle at the level of the umbilicus for larger ones (Fig. 2.42).

Scars of the abdominal wall near the planned flap contraindicate flap elevation. If a herniotomy has been performed, the forward flow of the inferior epigastric vessels must be assessed by angiograph. Hair can be a problem with a rectus flap, particularly for reconstruction of non-hair-bearing areas of the head and neck.

Flap Elevation

The flap is first incised around its circumference. A further skin incision is made from the middle of the lower edge of the flap over the rectus abdominis muscle as far as the lateral symphysis. The external oblique muscle is dissected epifascially from lateral to medial down to the rectus sheath, and the flap is elevated from the external oblique muscle (Fig. 2.44). The lateral edge of the rectus abdominis muscle must be correctly identified to avoid injuring the perforating vessels in the wrong layer of the rectus sheath.

The rectus sheath is incised parallel to the upper edge of the flap, along its medial edge to the linea alba, and parallel to the inferior edge of the flap. The rectus sheath is then divided along the lateral border of the rectus abdominis muscle, during which step several vessels must be ligated or coagulated. The rectus sheath is divided at the inferior edge of the flap above the linea semilunaris. After making a paramedial incision of the rectus sheath from the inferior border of the flap to the pubic bone, the rest of the rectus abdominis muscle is exposed inferiorly. The rectus abdominis muscle is divided at the superior part of the flap, after ligating the superior epigastric vessels. The muscle can now be removed from the posterior rectus sheath, during which several vessels arising from the muscle laterally and medially must be ligated and coagulated (Fig. 2.45).

The tendinous intersections are fairly difficult to dissect free of the fascia. Care is needed to remove the muscle from the rectus sheath without injuring the small vessels that run in the intersections. It is best to work from lateral to medial with a scalpel, with careful and immediate hemostasis. Next the inferior epigastric artery is dissected as a pedicle by lifting the muscle from medial to lateral out of the posterior rectus sheath; the vessels are then always visible and can be easily followed. They leave the muscle below the linea semilunaris. The muscle can then be divided beneath the entry point of the pedicle. The pedicle is exposed outside the peritoneum as far as the external iliac artery and vein. Before the pedicle can be divided the perfusion of the skin island must be tested; however, no tension should be exerted on the vessels.

Closure of the Donor Defect

When elevating the flap it must be kept in mind that in order to close the resulting defect, the duplication of the anterior part of the rectus sheath must be left intact to allow closure of the defect. Operating conditions are improved if the patient is given a liquid diet for several days before removal of the flap and the bowels are opened preoperatively. It is then easier to close the abdominal wall. We recommend leaving a suction drain in the rectus sheath donor site for 2 days.

The edges of the anterior rectus sheath are closed with a continuous suture secured by interrupted sutures at 5 cm intervals. If the fascia is successfully adapted, the skin can be closed without difficulty. An oval skin island that extends over the edges of the rectus sheath leaves a

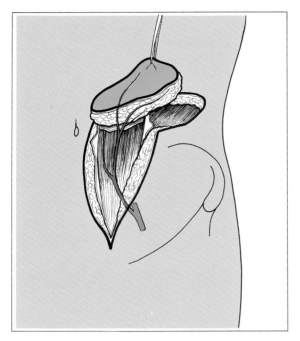

Fig. 2.**44**   First the flap is incised around its circumference. A further incision is made in the middle of the lower edge of the flap over the rectus abdominis muscle to the lateral side of the symphysis. The flap is elevated from the fascia of the external oblique abdominal muscle medially as far as the rectus sheath. After the lateral edge of the rectus abdominis muscle is exposed, the anterior rectus sheath is incised around the island of skin and from the lower edge of the flap down to the pubic bone.

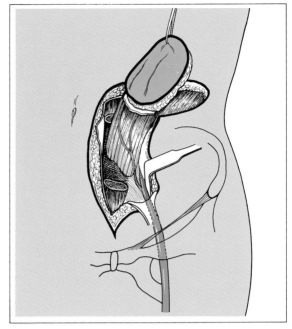

Fig. 2.**45**   The rectus abdominis muscle is divided at the upper edge of the flap, and the epigastric arteries are ligated. The muscle is elevated from the rectus sheath from medial to lateral exposing the pedicle, which leaves the muscle below the linea semilunaris. After dividing the muscle below the point of entry of the vessel, the epigastric vessels are followed to the iliac artery and vein.

defect requiring flap closure. Subcutaneous epifascial tissue is mobilized superiorly; the umbilicus may need to be excised and moved to a new site. The lowest portion of the donor site, where only the anterior rectus sheath is present, is naturally weak. Hernias have occurred at this site and we therefore recommend strengthening the posterior wall at the donor site after elevating the flap, for example, with absorbable materials such as Dexon mesh.

Monitoring the status of the rectus flap is facilitated, as with other composite grafts, if a skin island is present on the muscle. If the muscle alone is used as a transplant, it can be difficult to judge the vitality of its distal part. In the early stages it is often livid, due to congestion.

References

Boyd, J. B., G. I. Taylor, R. Corlett: The vascular territories of the superior epigastric and the deep inferior epigastric systems. Plast. reconstr. Surg. 73 (1984) 1
Pennington, D. G., M. F. Lai, A. D. Pelly: The rectus abdominis myocutaneous free flap. Brit. J. plast. Surg. 33 (1980) 277–282
Taylor, G. I., R. Corlett, J. B. Boyd: The extended deep inferior epigastric flap: a clinical technique. Plast. reconstr. Surg. 72 (1983) 751

Iliac Crest Graft

In the course of the development of free tissue grafts, an increasing number were found that could be used for reconstruction of bone, including a free fibular transplant on the peroneal artery; a second metatarsal bone transplant on the dorsalis pedis artery; a radial segment with a forearm flap on the radial artery; a free rib graft on the serratus anterior muscle or latissimus dorsi muscle with the subscapular artery or thoracodorsal artery; the scapular or parascapular flap with a bony segment of the scapula on the subscapular artery too; or the free iliac crest transplant on the deep iliac circumflex artery. Not all of these grafts have proven to be useful for reconstructions in the head and neck, in particular for reconstruction of the mandible.

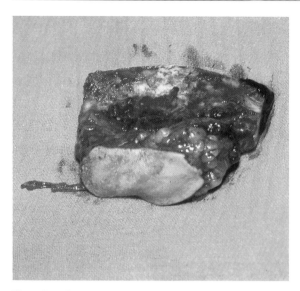

Fig. 2.**46**   Free iliac crest graft with a skin island based on the deep circumflex iliac artery.

In contrast to all the other above-named bone transplants, the shape of the iliac crest adapts well to reconstruction of the mandible.

The portion of the ilium that is available for free tissue transplantation is a 4-cm broad strip of bone harvested from the iliac fossa extending from the anterosuperior iliac spine along the iliac crest up to the sacroiliac joint. The iliac crest has an internal lip, an external lip, and a linea intermedia, which lies between them. The transverse abdominal muscle attaches to the internal lip and extends to the lateral third of the inguinal ligament. The internal oblique muscle begins at the linea intermedia, and it extends beyond the lateral half of the inguinal ligament. The external oblique muscle begins at the anterior half of the external lip, and its medial aponeurosis extends to the inguinal ligament. The sartorius muscle begins at the anterosuperior iliac spine; the tensor fasciae latae muscle attaches to the lateral surface of the anterosuperior iliac spine. The gluteus medius muscle extends along the lateral border of the ilium under the iliac crest; the iliacus muscle has its origin on the medial side in the iliac fossa and runs ventromedially under the inguinal ligament.

The iliac crest graft can consist of bone-bone, a bone-muscle, or bone, muscle and skin (Fig. 2.**46**). The transplant can be modeled from the relatively broad and flat bone to the desired shape. It is possible to achieve the necessary curvature of the bone by using a saw on the outside of the graft and stabilizing it afterwards with the help of a reconstruction plate. The good perfusion, generous amount of spongiosa, and stability of the transplant enable dental implants to be used later. Bone transplants with the overlying skin and portions of the sartorius muscle, the internal and external oblique muscles, and the gluteus medius muscle can be elevated, with the accompanying vascular pedicle.

Vascular Anatomy

Although the superficial iliac circumflex artery and vein are sufficient to nourish the iliac crest transplant, O'Brien et al. (1987) and Taylor et al. (1979) believe that the deep iliac circumflex artery is more reliable, particularly for supplying the bone. O'Brien recommends elevating the superficial iliac circumflex artery as well as the deep iliac circumflex artery when raising the iliac crest with a skin flap, because in 20% of the cases the skin area is not sufficiently perfused by the deep iliac circumflex artery. In our experience it has been sufficient to use the deep iliac circumflex artery alone as a flap pedicle.

The deep iliac circumflex artery measures between 1.5 and 2.5 mm in diameter and is 6–8 cm long. The vessel is much thicker than the superficial iliac circumflex artery. It is accompanied by large venae comitantes, which fuse to form one vessel that crosses in front or behind the external iliac artery before draining into the external iliac vein. The deep iliac circumflex artery arises just above the inguinal ligament from the lateral wall of the external iliac artery next to the inferior epigastric artery. It runs lateral parallel to and behind the inguinal ligament towards the anterosuperior iliac spine in the fascial sheath between the transverse abdominal and iliacus muscles, lying on the iliopsoas muscle (Fig. 2.**47**). At this point it crosses the lateral cutaneous femoral nerve. Lateral to the anterosuperior iliac spine the deep iliac circumflex artery gives off a large ascending branch, which can sometimes branch directly from the external iliac artery and run parallel to the deep iliac circumflex artery. At this point another vessel leaves the posterior wall of the deep iliac circumflex artery and goes to the iliacus muscle, which is often difficult to recognize. The deep iliac circumflex artery continues lateral to the iliac muscle and enters the bone about 1–2 cm beneath the iliac crest between the transverse abdominal and the internal oblique abdominal muscles.

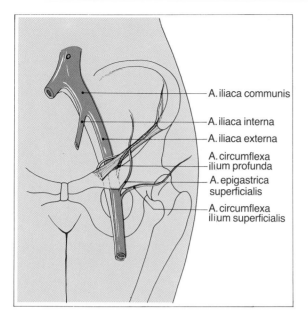

Fig. 2.**47** The deep circumflex iliac artery arises just above the inguinal ligament from the lateral side of the external iliac artery. It runs behind and parallel to the inguinal ligament laterally towards the anterior superior iliac spine.

A. iliaca communis
A. iliaca interna
A. iliaca externa
A. circumflexa ilium profunda
A. epigastrica superficialis
A. circumflexa ilium superficialis

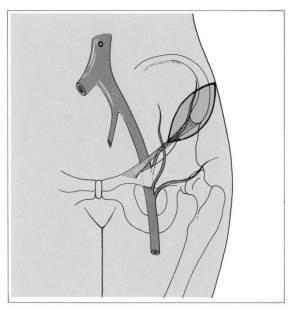

Fig. 2.**49** The anterior superior iliac spine, the femoral artery, the pubic tubercle, the inguinal ligament, and the iliac crest are marked on the skin.

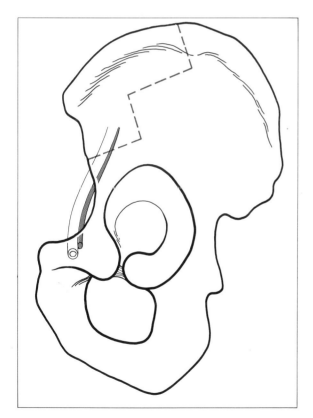

Fig. 2.**48** The bony segment of the flap can extend from the anterior superior iliac spine to the sacroiliac joint and include the upper part of the iliac fossa and the iliac crest. However, usually only the anterior part of the iliac fossa is needed.

Flap Planning

The available section of the ilium extends from the anterosuperior iliac spine almost to the sacroiliac joint, including the cranial portion of the iliac fossa and the iliac crest (Fig. 2.**48**). The skin flap can have a maximal size of 10 x 20 cm. Previous surgery in the inguinal area, such as herniotomy or appendectomy, can make flap elevation impossible, due to ligated vessels or damage to the perforating vessels. After the optimal size needed for the transplant has been ascertained by studying the receptor site, the outline of the flap can be marked on the skin. The flap is elevated with the patient in the prone position, so that it can be done at the same time as the tumor is resected.

First the anterosuperior iliac spine, the femoral artery, the pubic tubercle, the inguinal ligament, and the iliac crest are marked on the skin (Fig. 2.**49**). The middle line of the graft is marked according to the position of the iliac crest, so that the main axis forms a straight line between the anterosuperior iliac spine and the inferior angle of the scapula (Fig. 2.**50**). When drawing this line the skin of the abdomen must be stretched tight towards the umbilicus, because it can hang inferiorly over the iliac crest, particularly in older patients. If an additional skin island is to be elevated, it should be drawn symmetrically to

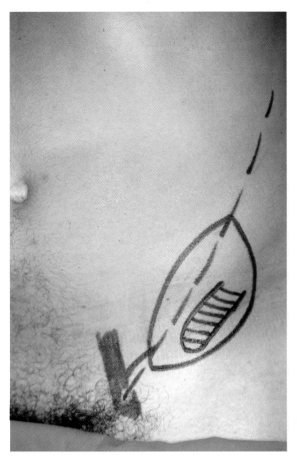

Fig. 2.**50** The skin flap is marked so that the main axis follows a straight line running from the anterior superior iliac spine to the inferior angle of the scapula. The cutaneous perforator vessels lie 1–2 cm above this line and 6 cm posterior to the anterior superior iliac spine.

the line already marked. The cutaneous perforating vessels can be found 1–2 cm above the line drawn and 6 cm behind the anterosuperior iliac spine; they should also be marked on the skin.

Flap Elevation

The removal of the flap begins with an incision around the circumference of the marked skin island. The skin at the upper edge of the flap is cut together with the subcutaneous fatty tissue as far as the musculature of the abdominal wall (external oblique muscle). The skin is fully divided over the fascia together with the subcutaneous tissue and the connective tissue layer from the fascia of the external oblique muscle towards the iliac crest. To preserve the perforating vessels, elevation of the skin should be carried no closer than 3–4 cm from the iliac crest. The skin must remain attached to a small strip of mus-

cle towards the iliac crest. Then the external oblique muscle can be divided just above the exposed connection to the subcutaneous tissue. A strip of muscle 3–4 cm broad remains on the iliac crest. Next, the internal oblique and transverse muscles are divided at the same level (Fig. 2.**51**).

The strip composed of the three muscles near the iliac crest should be at least 3–4 cm broad; in it lie the deep iliac circumflex artery and the perforating vessels. After incising the transverse fascia, the extraperitoneal fatty tissue is pushed aside by retracting the peritoneal sac medially and superiorly. It is now possible to expose the transition to the fascia of the iliacus muscle. The deep iliac circumflex artery can be palpated at this point. Then the subcutaneous tissue is divided as far as the tensor fasciae latae on the inferior border of the flap, and the fascia of the muscle is incised at its point of attachment to the bone; the tensor fasciae latae and the gluteus medius are separated from the outer surface of the ilium. The pedicle is identified and exposed through a skin incision above the inguinal ligament. All layers of the abdominal wall are now divided 1 cm above and parallel to the inguinal ligament and the fibrous connective tissue lying anteriorly is removed to reach the external iliac artery and vein.

Just above the inguinal ligament lies the deep iliac circumflex artery that nourishes the iliac crest, next to the deep epigastric vessels on the anterolateral side of the external iliac artery. Sometimes it arises from the external iliac artery on the same stem as the deep epigastric artery. The veins that result from the anastomosis of both venae comitantes cross in front or behind the external iliac artery, and drain into the external iliac vein, which lies medial to it. The pedicle is then dissected from medial to lateral as far as the anterosuperior iliac spine, and the ascending vessel branches and those for the iliacus muscle are divided. The lateral cutaneous femoral nerve must be dissected free from the vascular bundle. After the contents of the abdominal space have been retracted, the iliacus muscle is exposed and the deep iliac circumflex artery, which is palpable 2 cm inferiorly, is divided without injury to the pedicle. The muscle is pushed inferiorly from the internal surface of the ilium in order to reach the iliac fossa. Bleeding vessels on the incised edges of the muscle must be carefully coagulated. The bone is now exposed on the lateral and medial side beneath the iliac crest, and the segment needed for reconstruction can be

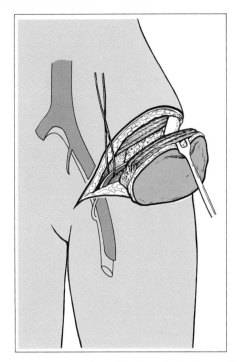

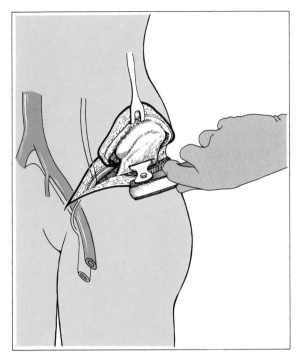

Fig. 2.**51**   After the skin island has been incised around its circumference, the three abdominal muscles are divided successively, so that a 3–4 cm wide muscle strip that incorporates the deep iliac circumflex artery and the perforator vessels remains attached to the entire length of the iliac crest. Just above the inguinal ligament on the anterior lateral side of the external iliac artery lies the deep circumflex iliac artery that nourishes the iliac crest.

Fig. 2.**52**   The bony segment can be removed with an oscillating saw after elevating the iliac muscle from the internal surface, the tensor fasciae latae and the gluteus medius muscles from the external surface, and the sartorius muscle from the anterior edge.

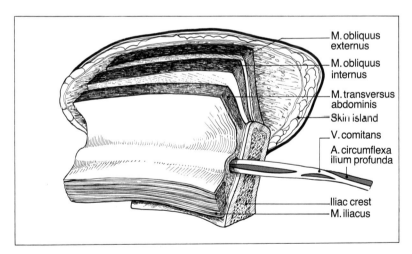

Fig. 2.**53**   The elevated iliac crest graft with all the tissue layers.

M. obliquus externus
M. obliquus internus
M. transversus abdominis
Skin island
V. comitans
A. circumflexa ilium profunda
Iliac crest
M. iliacus

marked off using a template. The bone segment is cut (Fig. 2.**52**) with an oscillating saw working from lateral to medial. The saw must be carefully watched on the medial side of the bone to avoid injury to the deep iliac circumflex artery.

When the bone segment has been elevated and the transplant remains attached only by its pedicle, the perfusion of the skin island can be ascer-

tained. If the pedicle is intact, blood should seep out of the spongiosa and the skin should have a pink color. The pedicle is then divided in the usual way; the artery is cut first and then the vein. The graft consists of a segment of bone from the iliac crest with a layer of muscle and a skin island of varying size (Fig. 2.**53**).

The iliac crest graft can also be elevated on the

superficial epigastric artery and vein of the groin flap, which arise under the inguinal ligament. However, this flap should only be used in exceptional cases, because of the irregularity of the vessels, their small diameter, and the poorer perfusion they provide.

Closure of the Donor Defect

It is particularly important to reconstruct the abdominal wall so that it is capable of bearing stress; the medial region of the donor site is subject to hernia development. The divided muscle attachments must be refixed with sutures to the pelvis or fascia, similar to the repair of an inguinal hernia.

The transverse fascia is sutured to the fascia over the iliac muscle. Furthermore, external and internal oblique muscles are sutured to the iliac muscle on the inside and to the gluteus medius and tensor fasciae latae muscles on the outside of the ilium. If the skin island is smaller than 8–10 cm it is usually possible to close the donor defect primarily. Otherwise a mesh graft of split skin is necessary.

References

O'Brien, B. McC., W. A. Morrison: Reconstructive Microsurgery. Churchill-Livingstone, Edinburgh 1987 (pp. 246–248)
Taylor, G. I.: Reconstruction of the mandible with free composite iliac bone grafts. Ann. plast. Surg. 9 (1982) 361
Taylor, G. I., P. Townsend, R. Corlett: Superiority of the deep circumflex iliac vessels as the supply for free groin flaps. Plast. reconstr. Surg. 64 (1979) 595, 745

Omental Graft

The greater omentum hangs from the greater curvature of the stomach; it consists of an anterior and posterior layer, and is freely mobile. Its position is quite variable: it can stretch over the transverse colon, hang in front of the coils of the small bowel in the lower abdomen, or be folded together in a small niche in the peritoneum. It varies in size, from a complete congenital absence to a size of 46 x 36 cm (Table 2.1).

Table 2.1   Size of the greater omentum (after Das)

	Men	Women
Length	25 cm (14–36 cm)	24 cm (14–34 cm)
Width	35 cm (23–46 cm)	33 cm (20–46 cm)

The omentum, together with numerous lymph vessels, plays a special role in immunity in the control of inflammation in the abdominal cavity. Its outstanding vascular supply motivated early surgeons to use it for reconstructive purposes. Its very large size allows defects to be covered that are hard to close with other tissues. Depending on how well fed the patient is, the omentum can appear thin and translucent, with little fat in thin individuals (Fig. 2.54) or full of fatty tissue in obese ones.

Vascular Anatomy

The greater omentum is perfused by two large vessels, the left and right gastroepiploic arteries (Fig. 2.55). The right gastroepiploic artery arises from the gastroduodenal artery, and the left gastroepiploic artery from the splenic artery, at the level of the hilus of the spleen. The venous drainage is similarly branched. Vessels connect the two sides, so that the omentum can be based on either pedicle. The main blood supply for the omentum usually arises from the right gastroepiploic artery. The gastroepiploic artery on the right is 2.5–3.5 mm, on the left, 1.5–2.5 mm. The veins always have a larger diameter than the arteries and they are thicker on the right than on the left. From four to seven large arteries branch from the gastroepiploic artery, course distally, and form a thick network of peripheral vessel arcades. Usually the arteries in the omentum are each accompanied by one vein.

Flap Elevation

The abdomen is opened through an upper median incision and, after placement of a retractor, the omentum is palpated for adhesions. Adhesions, particularly those resulting from previous operations, should be carefully separated, and only then can the further dissection take place. The omentum is pulled away from the transverse colon towards the abdominal wall. The connection to the transverse colon is divided with sharp scissors; bipolar diathermy is ideal for adequate hemostasis. The courses of the right and left gastroepiploic arteries are not only easy to palpate, but can almost always be seen easily. The accompanying veins run parallel to the arteries as a rule. Sometimes the vessels lie close to the greater curvature of the stomach. In these cases the vascular connection to the stomach should be ligated using very fine ties.

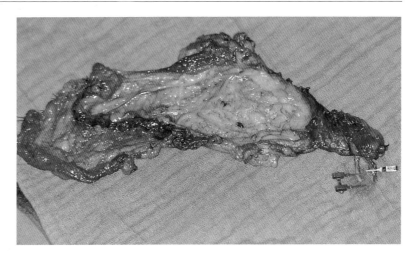

Fig. 2.**54**   Free omentum based on the right gastroepiploic artery.

How the omentum is to be elevated is decided during the operation because the degree and nature of its blood supply cannot be known beforehand. In some cases the right and left gastroepiploic arteries are directly connected to each other via a robust arcade, and either vessel may be chosen. The vessels in the omentum itself are very fragile. If they are injured, the bleeding must be stopped immediately. Bleeding blocks the field of vision and endangers the graft. For vessel injuries we use transfixion sutures of 5–0 nylon, which must be accurately placed. We dissect the last section of the pedicle in situ to prepare it for later microvascular anastomosis: during dissection outside the abdomen the relatively fragile veins are vulnerable. A donor defect does not follow elevation of the omentum. A drain is inserted and then the abdominal cavity is closed.

References

Arnold, P. G., G. B. Irons: The greater omentum. Extension in transpositions and free transfer. Plast. reconstr. Surg. 67 (1981) 169–176

Das, S. K.: The size of human omentum and methods of lengthening it for transplantation. Brit. J. plast. Surg. 29 (1976) 170–174

Jejunal Grafts

The coils of the jejunum fill the upper left part of the lower abdomen; the jejunum gradually merges into the ilium. The preferred donor region is the proximal jejunum. Terminal ilium can also be used, particularly when very long vessel arcades are needed. The pedicle may be dissected out relatively long if the segment of intestine lying directly over the vessel is rejected. Then it

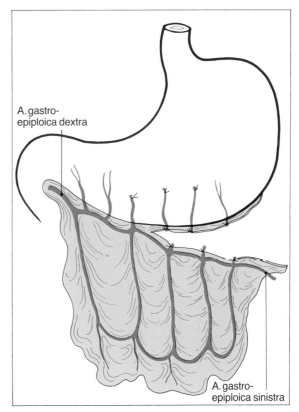

Fig. 2.**55**   The right and left gastroepiploic artery are usually interconnected via a large vascular arcade, so that the flap can be based on either side. The vessels to the stomach must be ligated carefully.

can be on average 10–14 cm long. The diameter of the mesenteric vessels varies, depending on the donor site; as a rule the arteries are up to 2–3 mm and the veins up to 4 mm wide. Meticulous hemostatis is mandatory during dissection. As with the omentum, bleeding in the mesenteric root obscures the operative field endangering the graft.

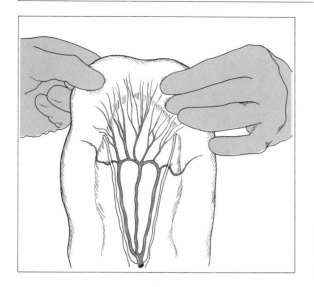

Harvesting the Small Intestine

A 20-cm long upper median laparotomy is made with an incision to the left of the umbilicus. A retractor is put in place and a proximal loop of the jejunum is pulled up. The transverse colon is pulled upwards with a liver spatula and the mesenteric root is inspected (Fig. 2.56). The vessels, particularly the accompanying mesenteric veins, are usually easy to see, and the artery can always be palpated. The pedicle becomes visible under transillumination (Fig. 2.57). The bowel is re-

Fig. 2.56   Careful inspection is needed to identify a suitable vascular arcade, usually lying in the proximal part of the jejunum.

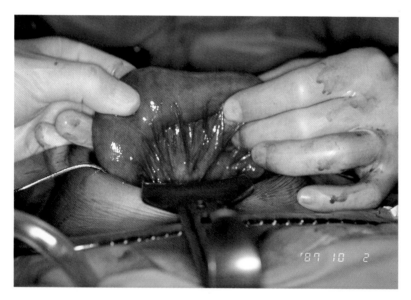

Fig. 2.57   The dissection of the vessels is made easier by transillumination.

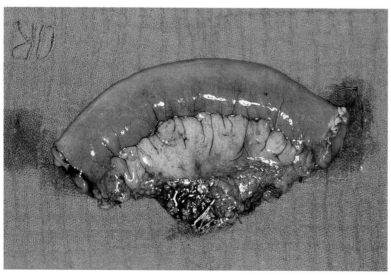

Fig. 2.58   Segment of the jenunum with a pedicle of normal length.

moved from the abdomen a segment at a time and inspected under transillumination with the help of an operating lamp, concentrating on the venous arcade and its main drainage. In this arcade the artery that supplies the corresponding segment of jejunum can be found and palpated.

After splitting the mesentery on both sides lateral to the vessel arcade, every mesenteric vessel that branches off is ligated and divided under transillumination. We try to dissect the last 2–3 cm of the mesenterial artery and vein macroscopically in such a way that anastomosis can be carried out easily. The artery is then clamped off before the vein. The mesenteric artery and vein must be handled very carefully. Deep transfixion sutures cause mesenteric venous thrombosis and should be avoided. A drain is left in place for 24 hours; we do not use heparin.

A clip gun is used to close the intestine on both sides and divide it at the same time allowing for a quick reanastomosis of the bowel to be done. Naturally, it is possible to suture all anastomoses by hand in one or two layers but a clip gun saves time, which is important in longer reconstructive procedures. The abdomen is closed after placing a drain.

It is unnecessary to store the intestine in any special way after its removal. Following short periods of ischemia, the intestinal lumen secretes generously after it has been reanastomized. Intestinal grafts that are first reconnected to a blood supply after only $1^{1}/_{2}$ hours react to ischemic injury with less secretion. This effect is advantageous in the reconstruction of the cervical esophagus. If a patch is needed instead of a segment, the lumen can be opened using diathermy on an already dissected arcade in situ. Hemostasis of the edges is achieved simply by bipolar diathermy. The length of the average pedicle is between 7 and 10 cm (Fig. 2.58). If a longer pedicle is needed, near-by vessel arcades can be included (Fig. 2.59), with the sacrifice of the neighboring bowel.

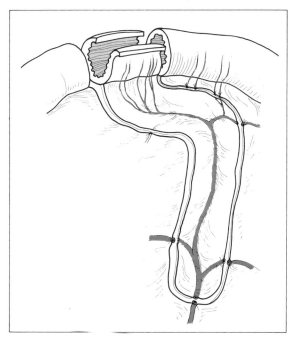

Fig. 2.59 **a** By sacrificing an adjacent section of bowel, its vascular arcade can be used to lengthen the pedicle.

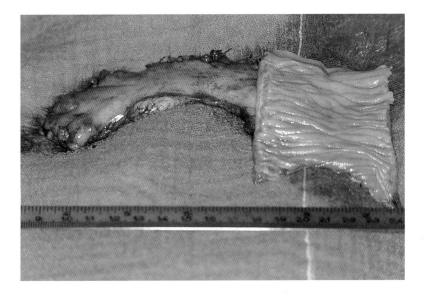

b Jejunal patch with a long pedicle.

References

Ferguson, J. L., L. W. DeSanto: Total pharyngolaryngectomy and cervical esophagectomy with jejunal autotransplant reconstruction: complications and results. Laryngoscope 98 (1988) 911–914

Flynn, M. B., R. D. Acland: Free intestinal autografts for reconstruction following pharyngolaryngoesophagectomy. Surg. Gynecol. Obstet. 149 (1979) 858

McConnel, F. M. S., T. R. Hester jr., F. Nahai, M. J. Jurkiewicz, R. G. Brown: Free jejunal grafts for reconstruction of pharynx and cervical esophagus. Arch. Otolaryngol. 107 (1981) 476–481

Renther, J., H. V. Steinman: Mikrochirurgische Dünndarmtransplantation zur Rekonstruktion großer Tumordefekte der Mundhöhle. Dtsch. Z. Mund-, Kiefer- u. Gesichtschir. 4 (1980) 131

Renther, J., H. V. Steinman, R. Wagner: Reconstruction of large defects in the oropharynx with a revascularized intestinal graft: an experimental and clinical report. Plast. reconstr. Surg. 73 (1984) 345

Robinson, D. W., A. Mac Leod: Microvascular free jejunum transfer. Brit. J. plast. Surg. 35 (1982) 258–267

Seidenberg, B., S. Rosenak, E. S. Hurwitt, M. L. Som: Immediate reconstruction of the cervical esophagus by revascularized isolated jejunal segment. Ann. Surg. 149 (1959) 162

3 Clinical Applications

Indications and Contraindications

Microvascular tissue transplantation plays an ever increasing role in reconstruction of the head and neck. The wide variety of flaps allows large and complex defects to be covered in one operation, facilitating a quick rehabilitation of the patient and reducing the amount of scar tissue of external defects that would result if local or regional flaps had been used. Nevertheless it should always be assessed whether a defect can be closed primarily, or whether a local advancement or rotation flap can be used without causing significant additional cosmetic damage. The disadvantage of free grafts is that the color and texture of the skin usually do not match the skin of the face, particularly when the flap is taken from the trunk. The great variety of flaps may make it difficult to decide which is the best flap to use. The surgeon who works with free flaps can hardly master the full range of grafts available, so that his experience with particular flaps plays an important role in the decision.

In choosing the tissue to be transplanted, the depth of the defect, its surface area, the need for bone, or internal or external coverage must be considered. The graft should be able to restore function and contour.

The ideal tissue transplant depends on the individual characteristics of each patient. For example, in choosing between a latissimus dorsi or a rectus abdominis flap, it must be kept in mind that the latter will be bulky in an obese patient. The defect must be considered, and the patient should be warned beforehand how large it will be. Some patients, particularly women, may find the defect on the volar forearm unacceptable. In these cases it is possible to use the dorsalis pedis or the scapular flap, but even the scapular flap causes a scar that inhibits women from wearing certain clothing.

Particular attention should be paid in reconstruction of the pharynx and oral cavity after tumor removal, so as not to impair breathing, swallowing, and speech. Thin fasciocutaneous flaps or free jejunum are available when superficial defects need to be covered. The movement of the tongue should not be significantly hindered by the flap. Some defects of the pharynx and oral cavity, owing to their extreme depth, must be covered with bulky flaps, which tend to limit function. In such cases, for example with multilayer defects, a patient sometimes must simply accept a functional impairment, but it should be kept to a minimum by choosing the correct graft.

The patient's age is not important in the decision to use a free flap but general condition and vascular status are. The oldest patient on whom we performed a microvascular tissue transfer was 81 years old. Vascular occlusive disease, arteriosclerosis, and hypertension can be relative contraindications. The risk of anesthesia and severe general diseases should also be considered, particularly for the laparotomy needed to harvest a segment of jejunum. In order to shorten the time under anesthesia in patients in poor general condition, a flap that can be harvested synchronously with the removal of the tumor and with the patient in a prone position should be chosen. In such cases the forearm flap is preferable to the scapular flap. Microvascular tissue transplants are always more time consuming than local or regional flaps. However, this is usually balanced by the fact that local and regional flaps demand several procedures.

Poorly healing defects, for example after radiation therapy and in infected wounds, are an ideal indication for a free flap, because the blood supply from the large vessels of the graft is usually better than average. In addition, the sympathectomy causes a dilatation of the vessels. This causes excellent perfusion, particularly at the edges, which is especially important for good healing of free flaps. Patients who have received radiation usually have poor vessels in the receptor area, particularly if the intima has been dam-

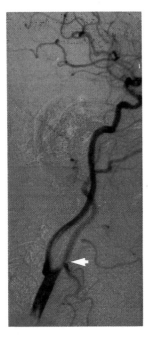

Fig. 3.1   In order to evaluate the vessels at the receptor site, subtraction angiography of the vessels of the neck was carried out 6 months after tumor removal. Only the superior thyroid artery (arrow) appeared suitable for an end-to-end anastomosis; the lingual and facial arteries had both been ligated at the first operation.

of arteriosclerosis and arterial occlusive disease in particular must be looked for.

The vascular status cannot be exactly ascertained by either angiography or Doppler sonography, but only by surgical exploration. Clinical experience and solid anatomical knowledge make evaluation of the recipient site possible. In patients who have already been operated on it is easier to find an artery than a vein for microvascular anastomosis. The veins are usually surrounded by scar tissue, and as a result, are more easily injured during dissection. It must be ascertained before operation whether the recipient site is suitable for the flap, as regards its depth and surface area.

Donor Site

The ideal flap combines good cosmetic and functional results at the recipient site with a minimal loss of function at the donor site. Scars due to trauma or previous surgery in the area of the donor site must be considered. Before harvesting a rectus abdominis or an iliac crest graft, a previous herniotomy or appendectomy must be ruled out on the forearm and dorsum of the foot. Previous vascular punctures must be considered. This is particularly true for the radial artery, which may have been punctured during a general anesthesia. Immediately before raising the flap it must be ensured that no superficial veins in the donor region are punctured: it is wise to mark the extremity to be used with the words, "no puncture." The flap could be endangered by a resultant thrombophlebitis. It is also important to ask whether lymph nodes have been removed or radiation therapy been given, particularly to the axilla and the groin, which could have damaged the vascular pedicle.

Damage to the region from which the donor vessel has been removed, that is, the hand or foot, can occur only with the forearm and dorsalis pedis flap. These flaps do not contain a network of end vessels, but rather those that pass through the region. Therefore it is important for both flaps that the perfusion of the adjacent areas is sufficient even after the donor vessel has been divided.

Doppler sonography is useful in some cases, to check the course and the forward flow of the vessels. Arterial occlusive disease must be ruled out. Allen's test should be carried out before the operation on the forearm, to see whether the perfusion of the hand via the ulnar artery through the palmar arch is sufficient (p. 21). This exam-

aged. This increases the difficulty of a microvascular anastomosis and increases the risk of a postoperative thrombosis.

Preoperative Diagnosis

In addition to evaluation of the general condition of the patient, the donor and recipient site demand assessment.

Recipient Site

It must first be ascertained whether vessels suitable for anastomosis are available at the recipient site. Abundant vessels are usually available in the neck unless surgery, e.g., a radical neck dissection, has been done previously. In such cases it is advisable to carry out angiography (Fig. 3.1) before the operation, to identify which vessels are still available. The venous phase should also be recorded in every case, because a thrombosis of the internal jugular vein can follow functional neck dissection. In addition, the general vascular status must be evaluated: signs

ination is usually sufficient. In questionable cases Doppler sonography and pulsoxymetry can be carried out.

To test the perfusion with the help of a pulsoxymeter, a measuring strip is attached to the thumb and index finger and the oxygen saturation is measured transcutaneously when the radial artery is compressed. A pulse curve can also be drawn. The pulse is felt over the dorsalis pedis artery if the posterior tibial artery is compressed and the pulse is felt over the posterior tibial artery when the dorsalis pedis artery is compressed. Only when the pulse can be felt in both arteries while the other is compressed, it can be assumed that both vessels are patent and have orthograde flow.

The flap must be measured before the operation to ensure that it is adequate to cover the defect. This is particularly important in the case of donor regions that have a relatively small surface area, such as the dorsalis pedis flap.

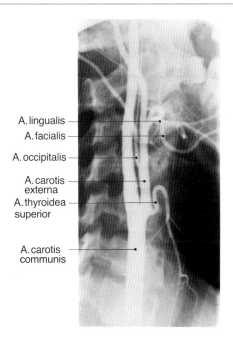

A. lingualis
A. facialis
A. occipitalis
A. carotis externa
A. thyroidea superior
A. carotis communis

Fig. 3.**2**   Conventional angiography of the vessels of the neck with imaging of the preferred receptor vessels (superior thyroid, lingual, and facial arteries).

Recipient Vessels and Preferred Anastomoses

The abundance of vessels in the neck is an ideal prerequisite for microvascular anastomosis. The head and neck surgeon knows the anatomy of the vessels well. During a functional neck dissection the recipient vessels can be simultaneously dissected, whereas in a radical neck dissection, they can be dissected on the contralateral side. The arterial vasculature available includes the external carotid artery and its branches (Fig. 3.2); we only choose the external carotid artery when no other vessels can be found.

The preferred recipient vessel for arterial anastomosis is the superior thyroid artery, because it is easy to find and is usually large enough. The anastomosis can be made directly above its origin from the external carotid artery, or more distal to it, if the donor vessel is smaller in diameter. The lingual and facial arteries also are available for vessel anastomosis. These vessels have a diameter between 1.5 and 2.5 mm. Incongruity in the vessels can be compensated for in the preferred end-to-end anastomoses by different techniques such as cutting the smaller vessel at an angle. The anastomosis is facilitated by use of approximator clamps. When preparing the recipient vessels the pedicle can be adapted whithout tension. It is always possible to make the pedicle shorter, but to lengthen it with vessel

grafts is not only time consuming, but hazardous because each additonal anastomosis increases the risk of thrombosis.

As mentioned above, all the vessels in the neck are not always available to the surgeon: often the superior thyroid artery may already have been ligated at prior surgery. In these cases alternative vessels must be sought. The anastomosis of the arteries is preferably carried out end-to-end with interrupted sutures, because a continuous suture tends to cause stenosis. When no other arteries are available, an end-to-side anastomosis to the external carotid artery is carried out. Frequently the wall of the external carotid artery is relatively thickened by arteriosclerosis, so that the anastomosis can be technically difficult to perform.

Only in exceptional cases, in which no other recipient vessel can be found and the external carotid artery has already been ligated or resected, should an end-to-side anastomosis to the common carotid artery be considered. In order to keep the ischemia time short, the anastomosis must be carried out quickly. The common carotid artery is taped and a bulldog clamp is placed proximally and distally. The adventitia is removed under a microscope using curved microscissors and the artery is incised with a fine pair of straight scissors. An oval defect is created

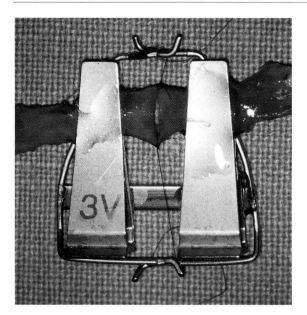

Fig. 3.**3**   A venous end-to-end anastomosis is simplified by attaching the angle sutures to the frame of Acland's approximator clips.

advantage of end-to-side anastomosis is the effortless adaptation of differences in vessel caliber. Even very small flap veins can almost always be satisfactorily sutured to the internal jugular vein. The internal jugular vein and the large facial vein can be partially closed off using a Satinski clamp, so that it is not necessary to expose and tape the vessel. We usually excise only a small part of the recipient vessel wall; here the danger of occlusion after a slit-shaped incision is significantly less than with an artery. For suture material we use usually 8–0 or 9–0 nylon.

We use approximator clamps for end-to-end venous anastomosis as well. They make it possible to approximate the vessel ends on the correct axis and to turn the vessel easier, facilitating suturing of the back wall. For this purpose Acland's approximator clips are useful because they have a frame that allows the vessel to be held by the long thread of the angle sutures (Fig. 3.3). Either interrupted or continuous sutures can be used; unlike arterial anastomoses, there is little danger of occlusion after a continuous suture of a venous anastomosis.

If the pedicle of the flap is too short to form an anastomosis without tension, it can be lengthened by using a segment of the saphenous vein. The saphenous vein is removed above the ankle, and turned through 180° to adapt the valves to the direction of blood flow.

The perfusion of the arterial anastomosis can usually be seen by the pulsation of the flap's artery distal to the anastomosis. If there is any doubt, Acland's test can help further. The vessel is occluded distal to the anastomosis by a jeweler's forceps, and a second forceps is used to empty the vessel towards the flap. Then the first forceps is opened: if the vessel fills immediately, the anastomosis is patent. The functional efficacy of the venous anastomosis can be tested by leaving the clip on the recipient vein closed while all other clips are opened. The circulation is thus impeded proximal to the venous anastomosis only. If the recipient vessel fills between the anastomosis and clip, the vein is patent.

Preparation of the Recipient Site

Two teams can often work synchronously in free tissue transplantation, so that the recipient area can be prepared while the flap is being elevated. The surgeon who removes the tumor can adhere to the principles of surgical oncology without fear of creating a defect that cannot be closed. Before the reconstruction, bleeding at the recipi-

in the vessel wall with button micro-scissors to ensure patency of the anastomosis. A slit-shaped incision carries the danger of stenosis and resulting thrombosis. It is not possible to suture intima to intima of vessels that have such a different wall thickness. The intima of the small vessel lies on the media or the externa of the carotid artery. For interrupted sutures, suture material of 8–0 is preferred to 9–0.

The venous anastomosis should preferably be to the deep venous system, either directly to the internal jugular vein or to neighbouring veins draining into it. The superficial venous system of the anterior or external jugular vein is indeed available but venous congestion can be caused by edema or a hematoma following the operation. This can endanger the flap. Another hazard is that the vessel might be damaged if a tracheotomy is necessary at the end of the operation. The drainage of the deep venous system is better and less affected by the development of edema and hematomas. If the venous anastomosis cannot be carried out directly to the internal jugular vein, it must be ensured that the chosen vein has not already been ligated at another point.

The more difficult venous anastomosis is usually performed end-to-side. The donor vein is held open by using the two angle sutures, making the further suturing of the thin vessel wall easier. A continuous suture can be used on both sides, starting from the angle sutures. A further

ent site must be carefully controlled; bleeding can elevate the graft, kinking its vessels. It can also be a nuisance during microvascular anastomosis. The recipient site should be prepared carefully, even when this takes time. This lost time is usually compensated for by a quicker anastomosis under good vision. The recipient vessels should be so prepared that the vein and artery lie close together, to avoid unnecessary separation of the flap vessels, and furthermore that they are easy of access and lie close to the surface, to ensure a tension-free anastomosis. If an approximator clip is used, it should be possible to turn the clip without hindrance. Suction drains should not be placed on the pedicle, but a Penrose drain should be used instead.

Reconstruction of the Oral Cavity and the Oropharynx

The incidence of carcinoma of the pharynx and oral cavity has increased considerably in the last few years. An increasing number of relatively young individuals between 40 and 50 years of age are affected. The demands placed on the surgeon who is confronted with an extensive tumor have accordingly increased. Because radiation is not indicated as the primary therapy in many cases, surgery has become more and more important. It is usually not possible to close primarily the defect arising from excision of the tumor, as this would cause functional impairment and reduce the patient's quality of life.

Therefore closure of the defect is usually necessary, after tumor excision, preferably using microvascular tissue transplants, because of their versatility, as well as regional flaps, such as the pectoralis major or the deltopectoral flap. Free microvascular transplants have the advantage that they can be sutured easily into every region, especially the soft palate, whereas pedicled flaps, such as the pectoralis major flap, can only be used at that site with difficulty because the pedicle is too short. If the mandible is maintained after tumor excision, the muscular portion of the flap (for example, the pectoralis flap) is often too large to lie behind the mandible in the mouth.

Fasciocutaneous and myocutaneous flaps as well as small bowel loops are available as free grafts for reconstruction in the oral cavity and oropharynx. The choice of flap depends on the defect left after tumor excision. If only the contour of the pharynx or oral cavity needs to be

rebuilt and the mandible can be retained, very thin fasciocutaneous flaps or a segment of small bowel divided along its antimesenteric border can be used. The choice of fasciocutaneous flaps lies between a groin, a dorsalis pedis, and a forearm flap. The groin flap is relatively thick with a short pedicle, which makes it unsuitable, so that we recommend either the forearm or dorsalis pedis flaps.

The dorsalis pedis flap is more difficult to elevate than the forearm flap because of the variability of the course of its vessels. Furthermore its size is limited to the surface area of the individual foot dorsum. Postoperative problems at the donor site are considerable: it is usually necessary to immobilize the patient for 10 days, which can lead to complications with older patients. Therefore our first choice is the forearm flap, which is comparatively easy to elevate and has a reliable and long pedicle. Rarely, we use the dorsalis pedis flap (Fig. 3.4) if for functional, cosmetic, and anatomical reasons the donor site appears more favorable, or if permission to use the forearm flap has been refused by a patient.

For the forearm flap we prefer the distal and the volar surface of the forearm, because this area usually has little hair. The thin and smooth flap with a relatively large artery in a long pedicle heals almost as well as mucous membrane and usually achieves a good functional result (Fig. 3.5). The functional results of reconstruction of the oropharynx including the soft palate and the inside of the cheek are better than those of the floor of the mouth and the anterior part of the tongue (Fig. 3.6). In the latter area we have observed swelling of the forearm flap in several cases that receded slowly after several weeks.

After the transplantation the keratinized squamous epithelium of the fasciocutaneous flap becomes converted gradually to nonkeratinized squamous epithelium, demonstrated by biopsy 1 to 2 years after the operation.

An alternative to the forearm flap is the jejunal patch (Fig. 3.7), which is preferred by some authors. Harvesting of a small intestinal segment is more difficult than elevating the forearm flap, and may cause more complications. This must be considered particularly in patients with cancer of the head and neck, because of their poor general condition. As far as the functional results are concerned there is no significant difference. When patients with cancer of the oral cavity and oropharynx receive postoperative radiation therapy, which they almost always do, the initial secretion of the jejunum, whose goblet cells are

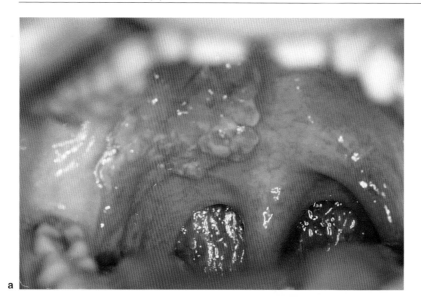

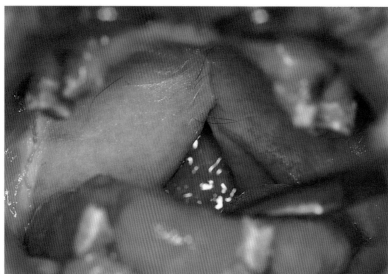

Fig. 3.**4** **a** Carcinoma of the soft palate, which has recurred after radiation therapy. **b** Reconstruction of the soft palate on the right with a dorsalis pedis flap after resection of the carcinoma.

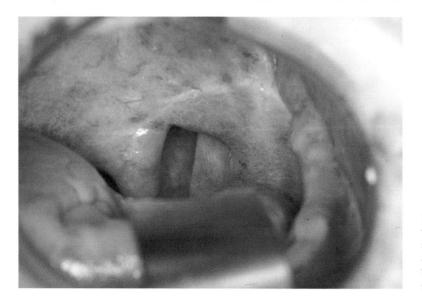

Fig. 3.**5** Reconstruction of the lateral wall of the oropharynx and the lateral soft palate with a distal forearm flap after resection of a carcinoma of the tonsils. Appearance 1 year after surgery and radiation therapy.

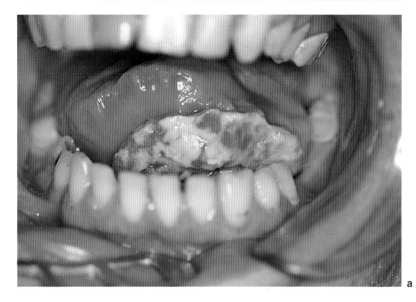

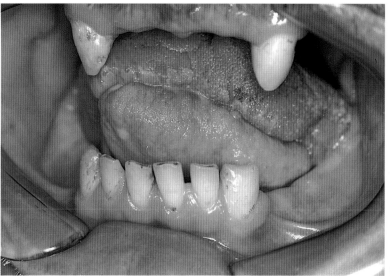

Fig. 3.**6**   **a** Extensive carcinoma of the anterior floor of the mouth and body of the tongue. **b** Appearance of the mouth after reconstruction with a distal forearm flap followed by resection of the carcinoma and dental attention. 6 months after the operation and radiation therapy.

already damaged by ischemia, ceases. After radiation therapy the graft is often observed to retract (Fig. 3.7c). The small intestinal mucosa is more vulnerable than the cutis and tends to bleed, for example, due to mechanical irritation from the teeth. It offers a poorer surface for dentures over the alveolar ridge than a fasciocutaneous transplant. In reconstruction of the soft palate the fasciocutaneous flap (Fig. 3.8) is preferred to the free jejunum, because unlike the jejunum it scarcely shrinks. When using the free jejunum there is a danger that rhinolalia aperta and nasal regurgitation will develop.

After extensive tumor resection of the floor of the mouth and the tongue very large flaps may be needed for reconstruction. For this purpose myocutaneous flaps are suitable, such as a latissimus dorsi or a rectus abdominis flap. The latissimus dorsi flap can be harvested in the appropriate shape with a small skin island and a large segment of muscle, so that the skin resurfaces the tongue and the muscle supplements the floor of the mouth (Fig. 3.**9**).

The free tissue transfer is particularly well suited for difficult transplantation sites, for example infected or irradiated areas in which local tissue cannot be used to close the defect. Free microvascular grafts have above-average perfusion even at the edges. One patient, who had no recurrence 7 years after excision of a carcinoma of

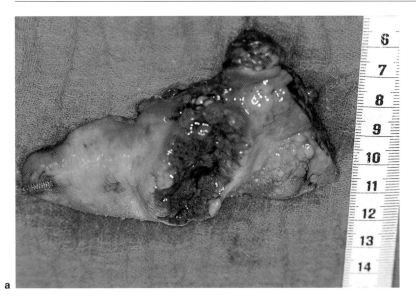

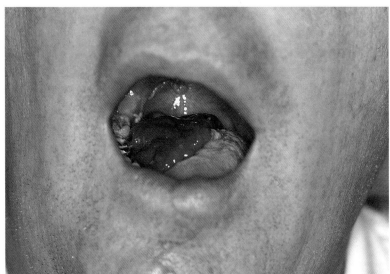

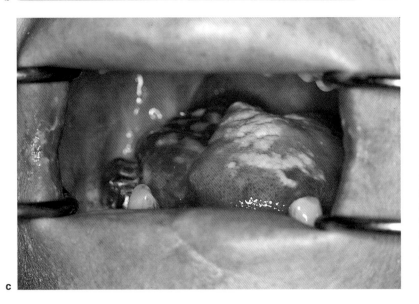

Fig. 3.7   **a** Carcinoma of the tongue on the right side. **b** Complete reconstruction of the body of the tongue after resection of the carcinoma with a jejunal patch. Appearance weeks after the operation, before radiation therapy.
c After irradiation the transplant has retracted.

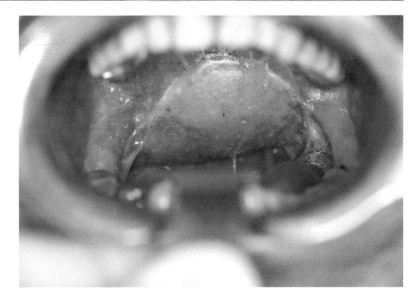

Fig. 3.**8** Reconstruction of the soft palate with a distal forearm flap after removal of a squamous cell carcinoma. Appearance 3 months after the operation and radiation therapy.

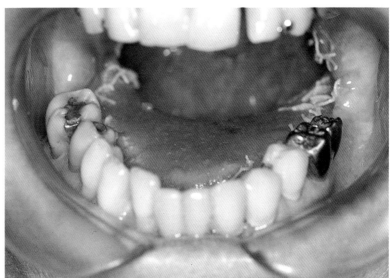

Fig. 3.**9** **a** Latissimus dorsi flap for reconstruction of the tongue.

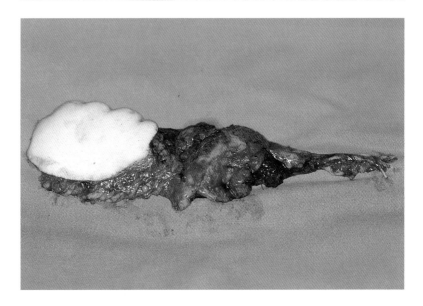

b Latissimus dorsi flap with a small skin island on a large segment of muscle.

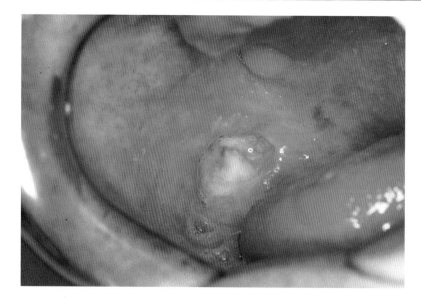

Fig. 3.**10** **a** A radiation ulcer that developed in the mucous membrane of the cheek 7 years after radiation therapy for a carcinoma of the tonsils.

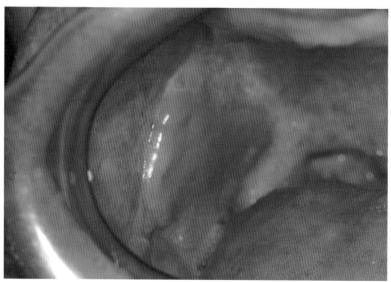

b Appearance 6 months after repair.

the tonsils, developed a radiation ulcer in the mucosa of the cheek (Fig. 3.**10a**). A very small flap from the distal forearm was used to reconstruct the inside of the cheek (Fig. 3.**10b**).

Very large grafts are necessary if a larger, multilayer defect needs to be covered as, for example, after a lateral mandibulectomy of a cancer of the oral cavity that has penetrated the outer skin. After a resection of the lateral ramus of the mandible, because of the minimal functional impairment we omit reconstruction of the bone, particularly for patients receiving radiation therapy. The latissimus dorsi or the rectus abdominal flap can be used for such cases. The fascia or a split skin graft sutured over the muscle serve as lining for the mouth. The rectus abdominis flap (Fig. 3.**11**) can be elevated together with the peritoneum and used to reconstruct the oral mucosa. The rectus abdominis flap is, however, not recommended for obese patients, because it would be too bulky. Also it must be borne in mind that the peritoneum tends to retract. Both myocutaneous grafts have a relatively long pedicle with a large artery and vein and so can be used for anastomoses in the neck.

All grafts mentioned can be elevated synchronous to tumor removal. The tumor surgeon must not adapt his procedure to solve the problem of

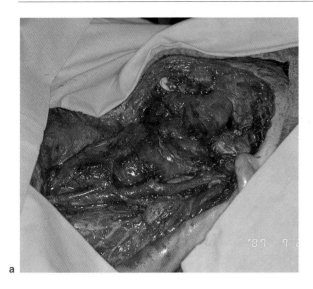

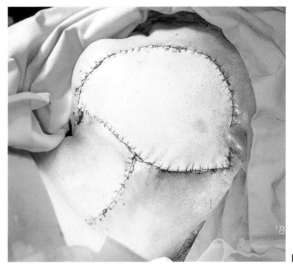

Fig. 3.**11** **a–c** Penetrating carcinoma of the oral cavity. Closure of a multi-layer defect that followed resection of the carcinoma (**a**) using a rectus abdominis flap (**b**). The lateral ramus of the mandible was removed, and the peritoneum on the inner surface of the flap was used to line the inside of the cheek. **c** Appearance 2 months after the operation.

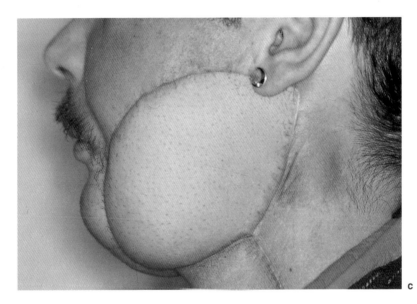

closing the defect but should carry out a wide resection margin. However, before the tumor is removed the expected dimension of the defect should be known, in order to plan a flap of sufficient size.

Before the vascular anastomosis the flap is brought into its ultimate position, taking care that the long pedicle is not bent or twisted. The pedicle is usually brought into the oral cavity or oropharynx along the medial side of the mandible, because it is the shorter and more direct route thus minimizing the danger of kinking or compressing against the bone. The access must be wide enough to avoid compression of the pedi-

cle. Careful hemostasis must be achieved at the recipient site, to prevent bleeding under the flap, which could elevate it and compromise perfusion. The graft is sutured in two layers to prevent dehiscence; the inferior margins are usually more at risk than the superior.

The wound must be bandaged loosely to prevent compression of the venous drainage. Circular bandages are dangerous as are retaining tapes for the tracheotomy tube; the latter is sutured to the skin.

Postoperative monitoring of the flap is often difficult, because the graft in the oropharynx is hard to inspect. The reasons for this include swelling of the tongue and the oral mucous membranes, pain, and lack of cooperation by the patient who is unwilling to open his mouth. In such cases fiberoptic endoscopy can be helpful.

References

Ariyan, S.: Pectoralis major musculocutaneous flap – a versatile flap for reconstruction of the head and neck. Plast. reconstr. Surg. 63 (1979) 73–81

Bootz, F.: Der freie Unterarmlappen zur Defektdeckung im Pharynx- und Mundhöhlenbereich. HNO 36 (1988) 462

Bootz, F., G. H. Müller: Microsurgical Tissue Transplantation. Quintessence, Chicago 1989 (pp. 53)

Harii, K.: Microvascular Tissue Transfer (Fundamental Techniques and Clinical Applications). Igaku-Shoin, Tokyo 1989 (pp. 144)

Manktelow, R. T.: Microvascular Reconstruction: Anatomy, Applications and Surgical Technique. Springer, Berlin 1986

McConnell, F., T. Hester, F. Nahai, M. Jurkiewicz, R. Brown: Free jejunal graft for reconstruction of pharynx and cervical oesophagus. Arch. Otolaryngol. 107 (1981) 476–481

Meyer, H. J., H. Terrahe, H. Haug, W. Schmidt: Die freie Dünndarmtransplantation zur plastischen Rekonstruktion von Mundhöhle, Pharynx und zervikalem Ösophagus. Laryngol. Rhinol. Otol. 67 (1988) 1

Muldowney, J. B., J. I. Cohen, D. P. Porto, R. H. Maisel: Oral cavity reconstruction using the free radial forearm flap. Arch. Otolaryngol. 113 (1987) 1219–1224

O'Brien, B. McC., W. A. Morrison: Reconstructive Microsurgery. Churchill Livingstone, Edinburgh 1987 (pp. 455)

Reuther, J., H. V. Steinau, R. Wagner: Reconstruction of large defects in the oropharynx with a revascularized intestinal graft: an experimental and clinical report. Plast. reconstr. Surg. 73 (1984) 345

Riediger, D., R. Hettich: Der mehrschichtige epigastrische Lappen zur Defektdeckung im Mund-Kiefer-Gesichtsbereich. Dtsch. Z. Mund-, Kiefer- u.a. Gesichtschir. 13 (1989) 203

Soutar, D. S., L. R. Scheker, N. S. B. Tanner, I. A. McGregor: The radial forearm flap: a versatile method for intraoral reconstruction. Brit. J. plast. Surg. 36 (1983) 1

Reconstruction of the Hypopharynx

The advantages of microvascular tissue transplantation are most obvious in reconstructive surgery of the hypopharynx. Formerly it was necessary to carry out several operations in order to reconstruct the hypopharynx with pedicled fasciocutaneous or myocutaneous flaps after a pharyngolaryngectomy. The patient was kept in hospital for several months. Postoperative fistulae often developed, and the patient generally had ugly scars on the thorax and shoulder. With the free tissue transfer the defect can be closed in one sitting, without significant cosmetic damage to the neighboring skin areas.

We distinguish between reconstruction of the entire hypopharynx and partial reconstruction with retention of the larynx. For partial reconstruction the jejunal patch and fasciocutaneous flaps, such as the forearm or dorsalis pedis flap, are suitable.

Extensive tumors of the hypopharynx filling the piriform sinus or infiltrating the larynx demand removal of the entire larynx and hypopharynx. The goal of reconstruction is to restore the continuity of the digestive tract by bridging the gap between the oropharynx and the cervical esophagus. The free jenunum and the fasciocutaneous transplant are both suitable. Harii discusses the use of the forearm flap as a fasciocutaneous flap for primary reconstruction. If the general condition of the patient allows, we prefer the free jejunal graft (Figs. 3.**12**, 3.**13**). When a laparotomy cannot be carried out owing to previous abdominal operations or other medical reasons, the forearm flap can be used for reconstruction (Fig. 3.**14**).

We always use an end-to-end anastomosis for joining the jejunum to the oropharynx, unlike Seidenberg who used an end-to-side anastomosis which often causes difficulty in swallowing. It also allows particularly high and wide anastomoses to be made. If the diameter of the intestine is less than the circumference of the upper section of the pharynx, the jejunal loop is incised along its antimesenteric border to widen it. There is usually no difficulty with the distal anastomosis to the esophagus. For this case we use a stapling gun to shorten the operating time. The lower row of clips is left on the intestinal segment, replacing the purse string suture. Usually a magazine with twenty-eight clips is enough. For incongruity of the apertures and a small esophageal opening, we use Gambee's technique of a single row of 3–0 absorbable sutures. Before the upper anastomosis is completed, the microvascular procedure is carried out, avoiding tension on the anastomosis.

When closing the skin we cut out a small window in the skin over the jejunal loop for monitoring the serosa, and thus the perfusion of the jejunum.

The defect in the skin can be covered after the fourth day with a split skin graft, for which the serosa is an ideal bed; alternatively, the defect will close spontaneously in time.

This simple technique for monitoring does not require expensive devices but is very reliable.

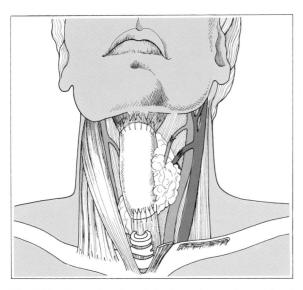

Fig. 3.12   Reconstruction of the hypopharynx by a jejunal loop.

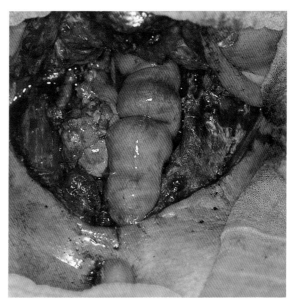

Fig. 3.13   Segment of jejunum used to reconstruct the hypopharynx after pharyngolaryngectomy.

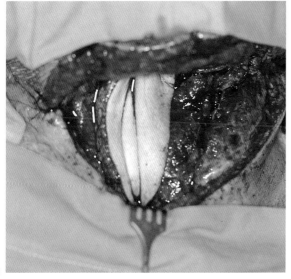

a

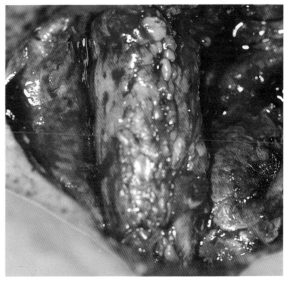

b

Fig. 3.14   Reconstruction of the hypopharynx with a free fore-arm flap after pharyngolaryngectomy. **a** The flap has already been sutured to the back wall of the oropharynx and the cervi-cal esophagus. **b** The forearm flap is tubed and sutured to the base of the tongue and the front wall of the esophagus.

If the forearm flap is to be used, a flap large enough to form a tube is elevated. First the posterior wall of the oropharynx and the posterior wall of the cervical esophagus are stitched to the flap with an inverted suture (Fig. 3.14 a). Then a tube is formed by suturing the anterior wall above and below, and the end of the flap closed on the anterior surface to form a tube (Fig. 3.14 b). Because the pedicle runs lengthwise in the flap and drains into either the upper or lower anastomosis, kinking of the vessel must be avoided at that point. This can be achieved by fixing the pedicle to the adjacent tissue with a fine suture so that a curve is already established.

After a partial pharyngectomy with retention of the larynx, the pharynx can be reconstructed

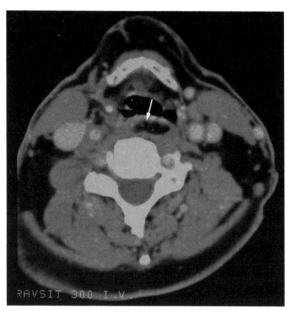

Fig. 3.**15**   CT scan of the hypopharynx. The back wall was reconstructed by a forearm flap (arrow) after the tumor had been excised.

using a fasciocutaneous flap such as a forearm flap (Fig. 3.**15**). A forearm flap can be used to supplement a stenosis of the hypopharynx after laryngectomy.

References

Bootz, F., G. H. Müller: Postoperative Überwachung des freien Jejunumtransplantates. Laryngol. Rhinol. Otol. 67 (1988) 606

Ferguson, J. L., L. W. DeSanto: Total pharyngolaryngectomy and cervical esophagectomy with jejunal autotransplant reconstruction: complications and results. Laryngoscope 98 (1988) 911–914

Flynn, M. B., R. D. Acland: Free intestinal autografts for reconstruction following pharyngolaryngoesophagectomy. Surg. Gynecol. Obstet. 149 (1979) 858

Harii, K., S. Ebihara, I. Ono, H. Saito, S. Terui, T. Takato: Pharyngoesophageal reconstruction using a fabricated forearm free flap. Plast. reconstr. Surg. 75 (1985) 463–476

McConnel, F. M. S., T. R. Hester jr., F. Nahai, M. J. Jurkiewicz, R. G. Brown: Free jejunal grafts for reconstruction of pharynx and cervical esophagus. Arch. Otolaryngol. 107 (1981) 476–481

Robinson, D. W., A. Mac Leod: Microvascular free jejunum transfer. Brit. J. plast. Surg. 35 (1982) 258–267

Seidenberg, B., S. Rosenak, E. S. Hurwitt, M. L. Som: Immediate reconstruction of the cervical esophagus by revascularized isolated jejunal segment. Ann. Surg. 149 (1959) 162

Closure of Pharyngocutaneous Fistulae

Fistulae are common after a laryngectomy but they usually close spontaneously within a few weeks. Fistulae in patients who have had radiation therapy are more usual. Some persist (Fig. 3.**16**), and must be closed. In particular, these patients have no acceptable local tissue for reconstruction since the perfusion, particularly at the edges of transposition flaps for example, is poor and healing in these regions is unreliable.

To close a fistula the myocutaneous pectoralis major flap or the fasciocutaneous deltopectoral flap have been used. The pectoralis major flap is reliable and simple to elevate, but its thickness and the resulting difficulty in modeling are a disadvantage. The deltopectoral flap is cosmetically unfavorable, and it usually requires two operations for its transfer. Free grafts are a useful alternative, particularly the double jejunal patch.

After a median laparotomy a 7–10 cm segment of jenunum is elevated. The bowel loop is divided between two arcades, so that both parts of the jejunum are nourished by a common pedicle (Fig. 3.**17**). Then the pedicle is divided and the two intestinal segments are opened along the antimesenteric border. The mucosa of one of the intestinal segments is dissected from the muscularis to prepare an ideal bed for a split skin graft. It is helpful to inject an isotonic saline solution under the mucosa in order to lift it from the muscularis. The entire mucosa must be dissected free very carefully. The intestinal segment with its mucosa on the inside is adapted using temporary sutures. Next comes the vascular anastomosis, which can be difficult after previous operations or radiation therapy. Because the superior thyroid artery is usually ligated on both sides during a laryngectomy, the anastomosis must use the facial artery or be done end-to-side to the external carotid artery. In some cases it may be necessary to use the transverse cervical artery for the anastomosis. The intestinal patch that has retained its mucosa is sutured in its entirety in the pharyngeal defect with the mucosa internally. The intestinal segment with no mucosa is used to close the skin defect, so that its serosa lies on the other intestinal patch. A split skin graft is laid on the exposed muscularis (Fig. 3.**18**). The split skin must be used as mesh graft, to avoid the development of a hematoma due to the good perfusion of the muscularis of the intestinal patch.

A fistula can also be closed with free omentum. The omentum has proven to be the ideal

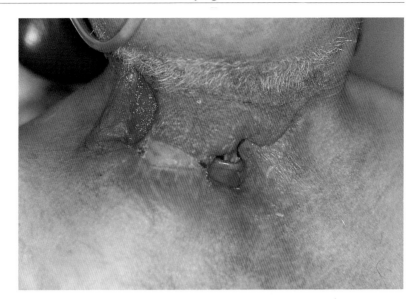

Fig. 3.**16**   A pharyngocutaneous fistula developed in this patient due to a pseudomonas infection after a laryngectomy. Initially the fistula healed spontaneously but it reopened after radiation therapy.

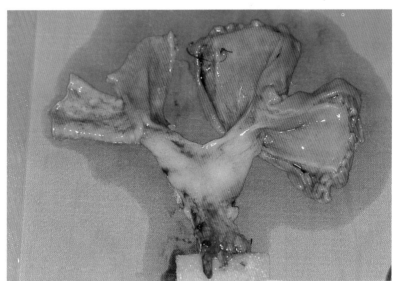

Fig. 3.**17**   Double jejunal segment, cut open along its antimesenteric border. The mucosa has been removed from the left-hand patch. The right-hand patch was used to reconstruct the front wall of the pharynx, the left to reconstruct the defect in the skin.

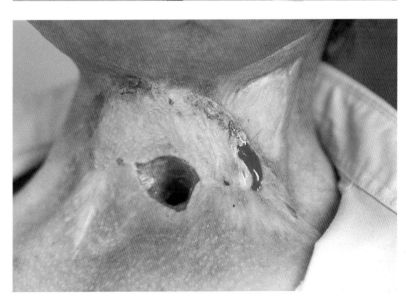

Fig. 3.**18**   Healed split skin graft on a jejunal segment from which the mucosa had been removed. A small residual area of mucosa that was not removed can be seen at the edge of the graft.

transplant in infected areas, due to its immune function. It can also serve as a bed for split skin grafts, so that it is possible to close large skin defects. The inner layer of the omentum is first sutured into the defect of the pharynx, avoiding overlapping of the omentum at all costs. The anterior layer is sutured to the edges of the skin and covered with a split skin graft (Fig. 3.19). The vessels have a long pedicle and a large lumen, guaranteeing a reliable anastomosis.

Free fasciocutaneous transplants are less suitable for closing pharyngocutaneous fistulae; free myocutaneous flaps are unsuitable.

These methods of reconstruction with free transplants should be reserved for those cases that have defied several attempts at plastic closure, or for cases in which it is known that healing will be poor, such as after radiation therapy or with chronic infection. For the patient who has been incapacitated for months or years by a pharyngocutaneous fistula, this operation clearly improves the quality of life, justifying the use of such an extensive and difficult operative technique.

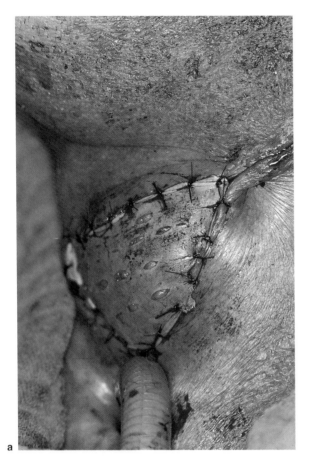

a

References

Ariyan, S.: Further experiences with the pectoralis major myocutaneous flap for the immediate repair of a defect from excisions of head and neck cancers. Plast. reconstr. Surg. 64 (1979) 605–612

Bootz, F., G. H. Müller: Repair of salivary fistulas after laryngectomy. Clin. Otolaryngol. 15 (1990) 299–302

Briant, T. D. R.: Spontaneous pharyngeal fistula and wound infection following larnygectomy. Laryngoscope 85 (1975) 829–834

Dedo, D. D., W. A. Alonso, J. H. Ogura: Incidence, predisposing factors and outcome of pharyngocutaneous fistulas complicating head and neck cancer surgery. Ann. Otol. 84 (1975) 833–840

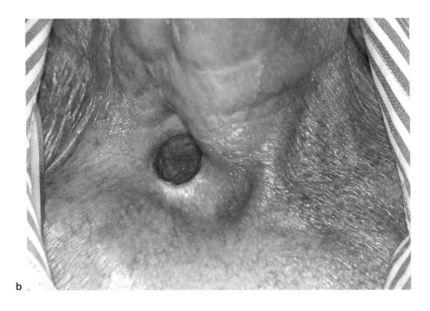

b

Fig. 3.**19** Pharyngocutaneous fistula. **a** Closure using a microvascular omental graft covered by split skin. **b** Results 6 months later.

Maisel, R. H., S. L. Liston: Combined pectoralis major myocutaneous flap with medially based deltopectoral flap for closure of large pharyngocutaneous fistulas. Ann. otol. 91 (1982) 98–100

Murakami, Y., et al: Repair of salivary fistula after reconstruction of pharyngoesophagus. Arch. Otolaryngol. 114 (1988) 770–774

Parnes, S. M., J. C. Goldstein: Closure of pharyngocutaneous fistulae with the rhomboid flap. Larnyngoscope 95 (1985) 224–225

Robinson, D. W., A. M. Mac Leod: Microvascular free jejunal transfer. Brit. J. plast. Surg. 35 (1982) 258–267

Stell, P. M., T. C. Coony: Management of fistulae of the head and neck after radical surgery. J. Larnygol. Otol. 88 (1974) 819–834

Reconstruction of the Mandible

M. Ehrenfeld

The mandible is a crucial organ for several important functions of the fascial skeleton.

- It serves as the point of insertion for the muscles of mastication, of the floor of the mouth, and of the tongue, and is particularly stressed in the act of chewing
- It provides the external framework for the attachment of the muscles of the floor of the mouth and the tongue, and therefore coordinates the act of swallowing and maintains the patency of the upper airways
- The mandible carries the lower row of teeth or serves as a base for a denture. In addition to chewing, the teeth, as well as the tongue and lips, play an important role in articulation
- The shape and size of the mandible determine the height and sagittal projection of the lower third of the face, and thus the aesthetics of proportion.

Loss of the continuity of the mandible impairs the aesthetics of the face and also chewing, swallowing, and speech. Parts of the mandible may be absent due to congenital malformation, but defects in continuity are usually acquired. Defects are caused by therapy of malignant and, rarely, of benign tumors or aggressively growing bone cysts.

Loss of continuity due to trauma or infection such as osteomyelitis or osteoradionecrosis is rarer.

Owing to the functional and aesthetic impairment caused by defects of the mandible, attempts have been made for over 100 years to restore mandibular continuity; alloplastic materials and homologous and autologous bone transplants have been described. A milestone was the beginning of free autologous iliac crest transplants in 1916 by Lindemann and Klapp. Today the autologous bone transplant is the first choice.

A bone transplant should be suitable in thickness, length, and shape to take over the biomechanical function of the mandible. It should be able to reproduce anatomically as closely as possible the different regions of the mandible in their curves and angles (for example, the chin and the angle of the jaw). These demands are fulfilled by the anterior iliac crest that offers enough material to restore mandibular continuity, though with a loss of height. Compared with free bone grafts these have the advantage of immediate perfusion, viable osteocytes, resistance to infection, a high perioperative antibiotic concentration in the transplant, and a volume that is well maintained. Also, free bone grafts can be used to fill long defects of continuity, as well as combined defects of soft tissue and bone. Thus they can be used in infected or irradiated areas, where free transplants carry a high risk of loss.

The biological properties of microsurgical bone transplants are always better than that of free bone, so that they are indicated also for areas that can accept a free graft and for moderately sized bone defects, to achieve the best possible reconstructive result. Owing to the longer anesthesia times required, the greater blood loss, and the larger wound area associated with microsurgical transplants, the biologically inferior free bone transplant is still to be preferred for a few patients in poor general condition.

Besides the iliac crest graft, several other microsurgical bone grafts have been described for mandibular replacement, for example the first metatarsal, the radius, the ulna, the scapula, the fibula, and the rib graft.

Reconstruction of the body of the mandible nowadays includes not only reconstruction of the shape but also aims to reestablish the masticatory function, usually by employing intraosseous implants. At present intraosseous implants have been described only after the use of iliac crest, scapular, and fibular grafts. Only the iliac crest graft always supplies enough bone to accept an intraosseous implant. It is sometimes impossible to use implants in the thin lateral edge of the scapula or the fibula. For this reason the iliac crest graft, also using microsurgical techniques, is the first choice for reconstruction of the mandible.

Microsurgical bone grafts are always com-

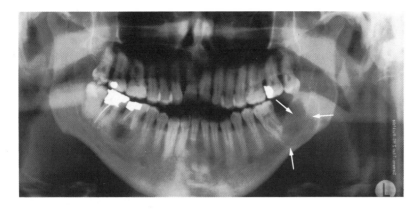

Fig. 3.**20**   Ameloblastoma (arrows) in the left angle of the mandible in a 39-year-old patient.

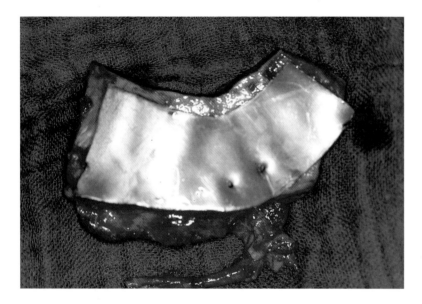

Fig. 3.**21**   Isolated osteomuscular iliac crest segment, that has been harvested with the help of a lead template defined by radiographs (same patient as in Fig. 3.**20**).

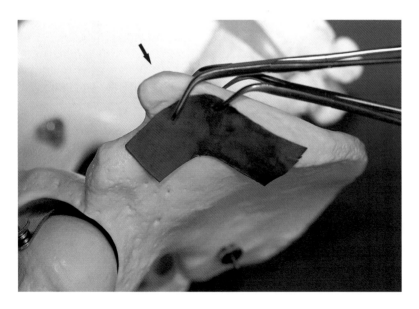

Fig. 3.**22**   The bone transplant that resembles the shape of the angle of the mandible is harvested from the iliac crest on the same side, so that the anterior superior iliac spine (arrow) forms the angle of the jaw (model).

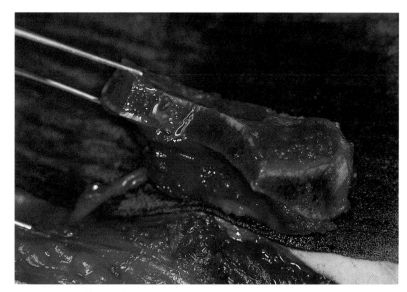

Fig. 3.**23**   An osteomuscular iliac crest graft based on the deep circumflex iliac artery and vein. The cuff of the iliac muscle can be seen in the extension of the vascular pedicle. The blood supply of the bone is delivered by the muscle and the attached periosteum.

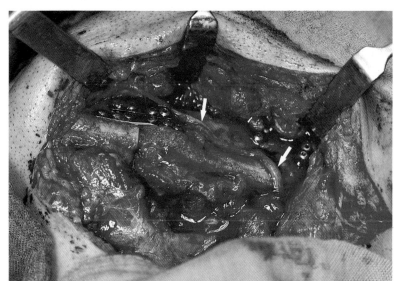

Fig. 3.**24**   An osteomuscular iliac crest graft that has been placed and fixed with osteosynthesis miniplates (AO plates). The cuff of muscle lies medially. The resected inferior alveolar nerve is reconstructed using a sural nerve graft (arrows) (same patient as in Fig. 3.**20**).

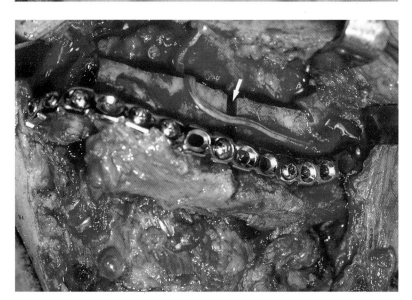

Fig. 3.**25**   If the cortex of a bone graft must be notched to bend it to the required shape, bridging plates (AO-reconstruction plates) are used for fixation. The arrow shows a cortical incision.

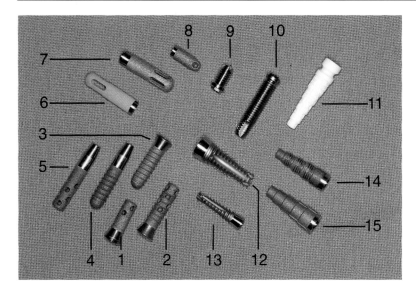

Fig. 3.**26** Modern intraosseous graft bodies offered by several companies in different materials and surfaces. 1–5: Titanium implant coated with titanium plasma from the Bonefit system. 6–8: IMZ implants; 6, titanium implant coated with hydroxylapatit; 7 and 8, implants coated with titanium plasma. 9–10: Brånemark implants made of pure titanium. 11: Tübingen implant made of aluminum oxide ceramic. 12–13: Titanium implant of the HaTi system. 14–15: Frialit II, cone-shaped titanium implants.

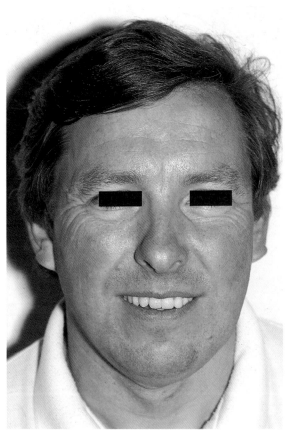

Fig. 3.**27** A 40-year-old patient 1 year after partial resection of the mandible and reconstruction with a free iliac crest transplant (same patient as in Fig. 3.**20**).

bined grafts of soft tissue and bone transplants, because a cuff of muscle and periosteum must always be attached to the bone. A paddle of skin can also be incorporated with grafts from the iliac crest, the scapula, and the fibula, so that composite skin and bone defects can be covered. This skin island lies at a defined place on the iliac crest and fibular grafts above the iliac crest or the contact zone of the soleus muscle with the peroneus muscles expertively, whereas a fasciocutaneous, scapular, or parascapular flap, can be elevated on the cutaneous end vessels of the circumflex scapular artery.

The advantage of these combined fasciocutaneous scapular–parascapular flaps and osteomuscular bone grafts from the lateral margin of the scapula is that cutaneous and osseous flap portions can be placed independently of each other (see above). The skin over the iliac crest has the disadvantage of being very thick if the subcutaneous fat layer is well developed, in which case it can hardly be used for intraoral reconstruction, unless it is reduced and thinned after the defect is primarily closed.

Primary and secondary reconstruction of the mandible must be distinguished. Primary reconstruction consists of a resection and reconstruction at the same operation, whereas in secondary reconstruction there is an interval between bone resection and reconstruction. Primary reconstruction is indicated in osteomyelitis and osteoradionecrosis, aggressive cysts, extensive benign tumors, and small malignant tumors. For extensive oral carcinomas (primary tumor larger than T1, suspect lymph nodes preoperatively), it

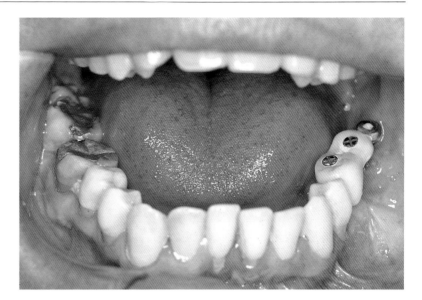

Fig. 3.**28** Same patient as in Figure 3.**20**, 1 year after the operation.
a Intraoral situation after partial resection of the mandible and free iliac crest graft: the transplant has been provided with three Bonefit hollow screw implants and a removable bridge.

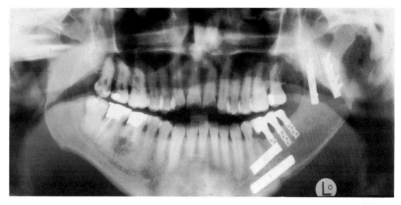

b Orthopantomogram after the operation. The iliac crest graft to the horizontal ramus of the mandible and the left angle of the jaw has been fixed with four miniplates. The graft has healed, and three dental implants have been positioned. The pelvic bone stands out due to its hypodense internal structure, in comparison with the thicker internal structure of the neighboring mandible.

is safer to reconstruct the mandible when no tumor remains after histological control of the tissue edges. Adjuvant radiation therapy should be carried out before the bone is transplanted to avoid osteoradionecrosis in the reconstructed bone.

Before primary reconstruction, the extent of the mandible to be resected is analyzed before the operation by radiology (Fig. 3.**20**), including computed tomography and possibly bone scans. Subsequently a lead template is made, which can be sterilized and used to cut the transplant to the required size (Figs. 3.**21**, 3.**22**). The iliac crest transplant is elevated from the same side as the defect.

A part of the anterosuperior iliac spine is chosen that resembles the angle of the mandible to be reconstructed.

Microsurgical iliac crest grafts should be based on the deep iliac circumflex artery and its accompanying veins (Taylor, 1979) because

these vessels provide more secure perfusion than the superficial iliac circumflex artery and vein (Fig. 3.**23**). The bone graft is fixed after securing the occlusion by an intermaxillary immobilizer (for example, jaw splints) using miniplates, because the graft needs minimal exposure (Fig. 3.**24**). The vascularization of the graft should not be compromised by too many unnecessary boreholes for the osteosynthesis screws. Vascularized bone grafts can be cut with a saw and bent after careful and discrete removal of the soft tissue from the cortical bone. If cortex must be cut and fractured, such as in restoring the chin, miniplates are indicated for stability (Fig. 3.**25**).

For future rehabilitation of masticatory function, intraosseous implants can be placed simultaneously or later (Fig. 3.**26**). We prefer intraosseous implants of titanium (for example, the ITI–Bonefit, Branemark, IMZ, or HaTi systems).

The prosthesis is fitted to the implants after a healing phase of at least 3 months. Microsurgi-

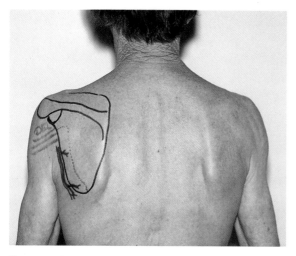

Fig. 3.**29**   Marking on the left scapula of a 61-year-old patient before a planned transfer of a bony segment of the lateral margin of the scapula. The bone is marked with a dotted line, and the position of its blood vessels have been drawn roughly.

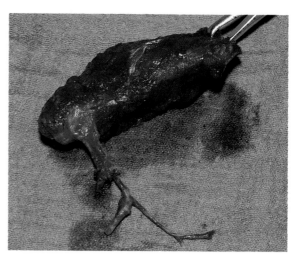

Fig. 3.**30**   Isolated pedicled osteomuscular transplant from the lateral scapular margin based on the subscapular vascular system (subscapular artery and vein and circumflex scapular artery with venae comitantes).

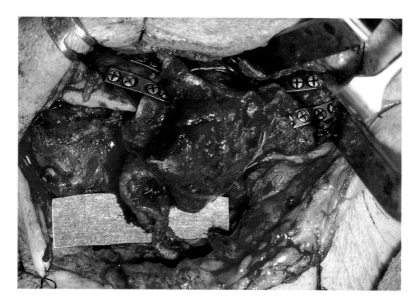

Fig. 3.**31**   An osteomuscular scapular transplant has been placed in the defect of the left angle of the jaw and fixed with four titanium AO miniplates. The anastomosis of the subscapular artery is carried out to the superior thyroid artery.

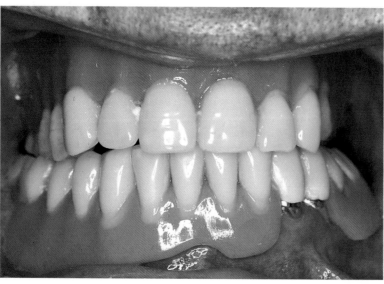

Fig. 3.**32**   Intraoral condition 6 months after bone transplantation. The transplant can withstand stress and the patient's mastication has been rehabilitated.

cal iliac crest grafts combined with intraosseous implants can achieve excellent functional and aesthetic results (Figs. 3.**27**, 3.**28**).

Secondary reconstruction often requires preoperative angiographic demonstration of the vascular topography in the recipient area. If satisfactory vessels are present, then the iliac crest is the transplant of choice. If a longer pedicle is needed, then the scapular graft (Figs. 3.**29**, 3.**30**) is an alternative, because its pedicle usually has a length of up to 13 cm, as opposed to 6–8 cm available with the iliac crest graft.

The advantage of the long pedicle of the scapular graft is balanced by the technical disadvantage that the graft is elevated when the patient is lying on his side, whereas the exposure of the receptor site and the placement of the graft are carried out in a prone position. This demands exact preoperative planning, so that the graft must be elevated at the beginning of the operation, in order that the patient need be moved only once during the procedure. The mass of bone of the lateral scapular margin resembles an atrophic mandible for purposes of transplantation. Owing to its well-vascularized cuff of muscle and its long pedicle, it is sometimes indicated, for example, for patients who have been already operated on and have received radiation therapy. The fixation is carried out after the occlusion has been secured during the operation. This can be done with dentures or a splint on patients who are edentulous or have only a few teeth, or those with miniplates, so that as little muscle as possible must be removed (Fig. 3.**31**). The functional and aesthetic results achieved with this procedure are good, although the angle of the reconstructed jaw is usually not anatomically correct because of the paucity of bone (Figs. 3.**32**–3.**34**).

Primary and secondary combined bone and soft tissue reconstruction do not differ from microsurgical grafts of isolated bone as far as the planning and execution of bone replacement are concerned. The area of the skin that must be transplanted is determined before or during the operation using a template (p. 72).

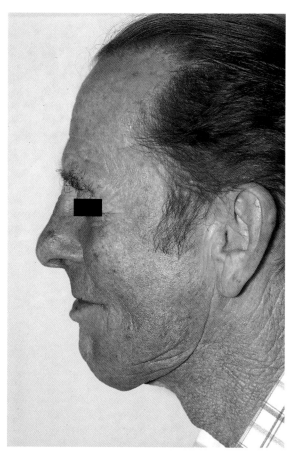

Fig. 3.**33**   Lateral view 6 months after reconstruction of the angle of the mandible on the left side and part of the ascending ramus of the mandible with a free scapular graft. The scapular bone does not exactly match the angle of the mandible.

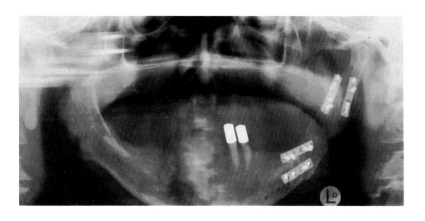

Fig. 3.**34**   Postoperative orthopantogram (OPT). The scapular bony segment has been fixed with four miniplates (Figs. 3.**29**–3.**34** same patient).

References

Ehrenfeld, M.: Die freie und mikrochirugische Unterkiefer-ersatzplastik vom Beckenkamm. Ein experimenteller Vergleich zweier Methoden. Habil., Tübingen 1989

Hidalgo, D. A., M. El-Tamer, T. Chaglassian: Aesthetic improvements in free flap mandible reconstruction. Plast. Surg. Forum 11 (1988) 122–123

O'Brien, B. McC., W. A. Morrison, A. M. MacLeod, B. J. Dooley: Microvascular osteocutaneous transfer using the groin flap and iliac crest and the dorsalis pedis and second metatarsal. Brit. J. plast. Surg. 32 (1979) 188–206

Richards, M. A., M. D. Poole, A. M. Godfrey: The serratus anterior/rib composite flap in mandibular reconstruction. Brit. J. plast. Surg. 37 (1985) 446–477

Riediger, D.: Restoration of mastatory function by microsurgically revascularized iliac crest bone grafts using enosseous implants. Plast. reconstr. Surg. 81 (1988) 861–876

Riediger, D., B. d'Hoedt, W. Pielsticker: Wiederherstellung der Kaufunktion durch enossale Implantate nach Beckenkammtransplantation mit mikrochirurgischem Gefäßanschluß. Dtsch. Z. Mund-, Kiefer- u. Gesichtschir. 10 (1986) 102–107

Sanders, R., B. J. Mayou: A new vascularized bone graft transferred by microvascular anastomosis as a free flap. Brit. J. Surg. 66 (1979) 787–788

Soutar, D. S., L. R. Scheker, N. S. B. Tanner, I. A. McGregor: The radial forearm flap: a versatile method for intra-oral reconstruction. Brit. J. plast. Surg. 36 (1983) 1–8

Swartz, W. M., J. C. Banis, E. D. Newton, S. S. Ramasastry, N. F. Jones, R. Aclanad: The osteocutaneous scapular flap for mandibular and maxillary reconstruction. Plast. reconstr. Surg. 77 (1986) 530–545

Tahara, S., T. Susuki, T. Kikui, S. Sagara: Mandibular reconstruction with subsequent denture implantation. Brit. J. plast. Surg. 42 (1989) 344–346

Tamai, S.: Iliac osteocutaneous neurosensory flap. In Serafin, D., H. Buncke: Microsurgical Composite Tissue Transplantation. Mosby, St. Louis 1979

Taylor, G. I., P. Townsend, R. Corlett: Superiority of the deep circumflex iliac vessels as the supply for free groin flaps. Plast. reconstr. Surg. 64 (1979) 595, 745

Reconstruction of the Surface of the Neck and Face

The surface of the head and neck can be reconstructed by local rotation, advancement, or transposition flaps, which have the advantage of color and texture match. More difficult situations require free microvascular grafts. Very thin fasciocutaneous flaps are well suited for the reconstruction of superficial defects, the forearm flap being particularly useful because of the ease of harvesting and its long pedicle. The dorsalis pedis and groin flaps can also be used but the former flap is limited by the area of the individual foot. The groin flap usually contains too much subcutaneous fat tissue and often has hair.

In reconstruction of burn injuries of the neck, as first described by Yang Guofan and coworkers, it may be necessary to use the forearm flap for functional as well as cosmetic reasons (Fig. 3.35). It is possible to use larger flaps that include almost the entire surface of the volar aspect of the forearm. The pedicle is then relatively short, but long enough for anastomosis to the superior thyroid vessels. Dissection in the proximal region must be carried out very carefully, as it is easy to cut the pedicle inadvertently where it lies in deep intermuscular fascia (pp. 20, 22).

After resection of extensive skin tumors where it is no longer possible to use a local advancement flap, a microvascular graft can cover the defect in one sitting without risking significant cosmetic damage to the neighboring areas, such as would be caused by a deltopectoral flap. If very broad and deep defects have to be closed after tumor excision, the bulkier flaps from the middle and proximal forearm area can be used. The smooth forearm flap adapts well to the skin of the neck (Fig. 3.36).

Postoperative radiation therapy can be performed after any free graft. Postoperative problems in wound healing are more frequent in irradiated areas. In this case the free forearm flap, with its well-perfused edges, offers ideal conditions for smooth healing.

Muscle flaps can be used for deep defects, the muscle being covered with a split skin graft (Fig. 3.37). The neurovascular latissimus dorsi flap can be used for the face, particularly facial nerve resection carried so far peripherally that it is no longer possible to perform a neural anastomosis. The thoracodorsal nerve is anastomized to a branch or main trunk of the facial nerve serving to innervate muscle on the affected side of the face.

The connection between the orbit and the nasal cavity and sinuses after the orbit has been exenterated for an infiltrating tumor of the cavities can be closed by free fasciocutaneous (Fig. 3.38) or myocutaneous flaps (Fig. 3.39). Recurrence of the tumor is better evaluated after the use of a fasciocutaneous than a myocutaneous flap, because it does not fully obliterate the orbit, thus allowing regular endoscopic evaluations to be carried out. Myocutaneous flaps have the advantage of being better able to close a CSF leak because the larger muscle mass obliterates the defect. We usually choose the facial artery and vein for anastomosis because the temporal vessels,

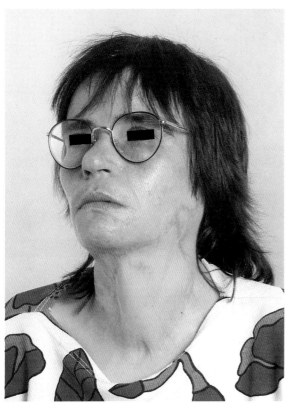

Fig. 3.**35**   Functional and cosmetic reconstruction of the skin of the lateral neck using a forearm flap to correct extensive contractures due to scarring after burns.

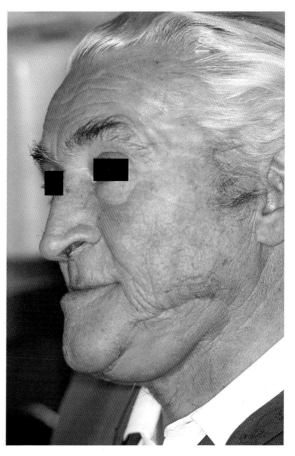

Fig. 3.**36**   Reconstruction of the submandibular area in the case of an extensive superficial defect, due to excision of a basal cell carcinoma, using a forearm flap.

particularly the vein, are unreliable, especially in patients who have received radiation therapy before the operation. A pedicle of 10–15 cm is needed to bridge the distance to the orbit.

A patient with a hemangioendothelioma who underwent a radical operation in which the middle ear was removed followed by radiation therapy 30 years previously, developed recurring inflammation of the mastoid cavity, which did not epithelialize, due to the radiation. Several attempts to cover the space with a local transposition flap failed. We inserted a small, distal elevated forearm flap with a long pedicle into the large cavity and attached it to the superior thyroid artery and the internal jugular vein. This was the smallest flap we had used up to that time.

This reconstruction is rarely indicated but the example shows that the forearm flap can be used in many different ways. A small flap is vulnerable owing to the danger of venous congestion

when the venous perfusion is not sufficient to accomodate the arterial load.

The cosmetic result at the site of the defect on the forearm is not always satisfactory, particularly in women; for this reason, the flap is rejected by some authors, especially when it is used for cosmetic reasons, such as after excision of a scar. To achieve a cosmetic improvement at the receptor site one must be prepared to accept a loss at the donor site. The scapular or parascapular flaps are alternatives to the forearm flap for the reconstruction of defects of the external surface of the head and neck. They have the advantage of a more cosmetically acceptable donor defect, because it can be closed primarily, but the scar often broadens. However, these flaps are often much bulkier than the forearm flap and thus limited in use. They are well suited for cases in which the defect must both be closed and augmented (Fig. 3.**40**).

Forearm flaps are indicated if a superficial de-

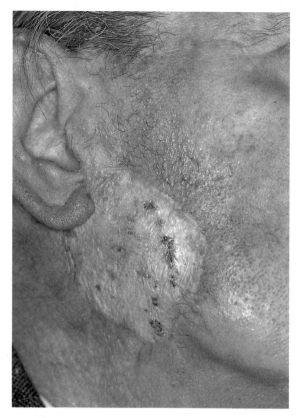

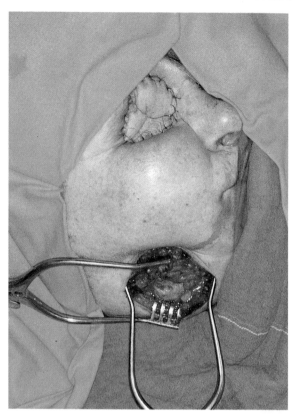

Fig. 3.**37** Closure of a deep defect of the face with a simple muscle flap from the latissimus dorsi muscle, covered with a split skin graft. Appearance 6 months after the operation and radiation therapy.

Fig. 3.**38** Closure of the orbit after orbital exenteration using a forearm flap, attached by a long pedicle to the facial artery and vein.

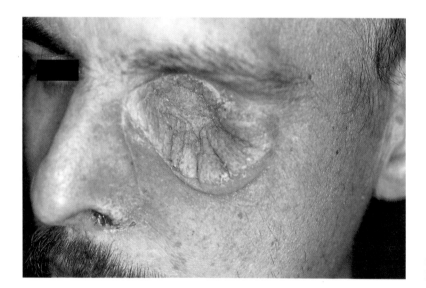

Fig. 3.**39** Closure of the orbit with a latissimus dorsi flap.

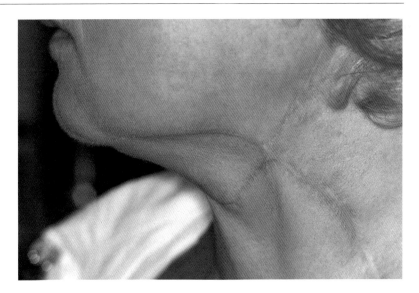

Fig. 3.**40**   Extensive deep defect after removal of a tumor in the submandibular region reconstructed with a scapular flap.

fect cannot be closed with local flaps, be it due to the size of the defect, the effects of infection or irradiation, or for anatomical constraints, such as in the orbit.

Myocutaneous flaps can be used for larger and deeper defects after tumor excision. Defects resulting from tumor excision that include several tissue layers including bone can best be covered with well-perfused myocutaneous flaps. The exposure of the brain after resection of the temporal bone and the infiltrated dura demands a reliable reconstruction, not least to prevent infection after the operation (Fig. 3.41). The latissimus dorsi flap is particularly well suited for this.

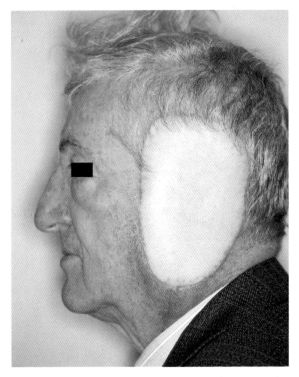

Fig. 3.**41**   Reconstruction after petrosectomy for an extensive infiltrating carcinoma of the auricle using a latissimus dorsi flap.

Augmentation for Facial Asymmetry
M. Ehrenfeld

Subcutaneous tissue deficits can be congenital or acquired. Congenital soft tissue defects of the face occur in mandibulofacial dysostosis (the Franceschetti syndrome), in which subcutaneous fat or musculature alone or in combination with bony sections of the mandible are absent. However, soft tissue defects can also be due to trauma, inflammation or surgical or radiation therapy for tumors. The etiology of progressive facial hemiatrophy (Romberg disease) is not known. The disease usually affects the middle third of the face on one side (Fig. 3.**42**). In most cases only the soft tissue is affected by the atrophy but bone can also be atrophic causing considerable disfigurement. The process of atrophy usually ceases spontaneously, so an augmentation should take place after the process has stopped. As a result of this tissue deficit the skin also shrinks to adapt to the underlying structure. Smaller contour defects can be corrected by a free transplant of supporting tissue (autologous or homologous cartilage, autologous bone, and in some cases alloplastic material) or by moving soft tissue from neighboring areas, for example, subcutaneous fat.

Extensive tissue deficits of the face should be managed by replacing the tissue with one of a similar texture. Large free grafts of fat are not suitable for this purpose, because they tend to undergo central necrosis, forming oil cysts. Microsurgery has made it possible to create transplants with good perfusion, viability, and constant volume. Compared with free grafts of fat, for example, they have the advantage of not undergoing shrinkage. However, this is not true of myocutaneous flaps, in which the denervated muscle atrophies.

Various microvascularized flaps have been described for this problem:

- Deepithelized scapular flaps
- Greater omentum
- Deepithelized groin flaps
- Axillary flaps

The groin flap has lost favor in reconstructive surgery; it is usually too large, but has the advantage of leaving no disturbing scar after closure of the defect. The vessels of the axillary flap have an irregular course like those of the groin flap, so that it is also only used in exceptional cases.

The omentum offers ideal characteristics for reconstruction of the contours of the face, although a laparotomy is necessary to harvest it. The omentum (p. 51) can be harvested in whatever size is needed in the individual case. Finger-shaped extensions can be developed to augment several areas of the face (Fig. 3.**43**). The omentum can also be folded, providing that its vessels are not kinked. These grafts must be fixed to their bed by percutaneous sutures, to prevent caudal sinking of the graft.

An alternative to the omentum, particularly when the patient refuses a laparotomy, is the deepithelized scapular flap (Fig. 3.**44**). This flap consists of subcutaneous fat with a deepithelized layer of skin above. The flap vessels have a regular course and diameter, which is an advantage. The elevation of the flap (p. 35) creates an easily visible scar, however, which can be disturbing, particularly for women. The scapular flap does not retract so that it is not necessary to allow for retraction in planning the flap. If the flap is too large after having healed, liposuction can be performed to achieve a better cosmetic result. As with all deepithelized transplants, the epidermis must be fully removed.

To establish access for most facial augmentation operations an S-shaped preauricular incision is carried out, similar to that for face lifts (Fig. 3.**45**). The anastomosis is almost always made to the facial artery and vein or the temporal vessels.

The omentum and the deepithelized scapular flap have become established as standard for augmentation in the facial region and because

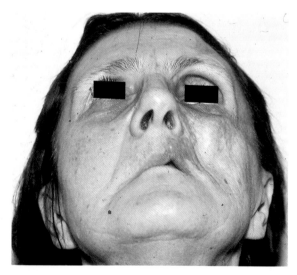

Fig. 3.**42** Hemifacial atrophy affecting all three levels of the face (forehead, cheek, and lower face) in a 59-year-old patient.

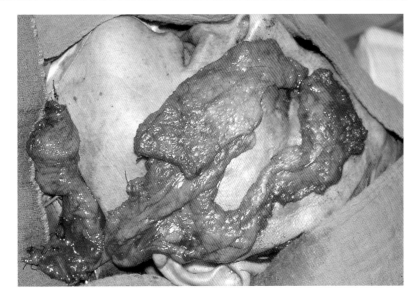

Fig. 3.**43** Greater omentum adapted to augment the left half of the face. The transplant is split and spread out so that it is possible to augment all affected areas of the face. The orbital fat can be supplemented also after lateral orbitotomy.

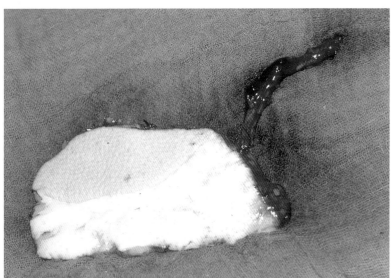

Fig. 3.**44** Isolated fasciocutaneous scapular flap, which is for the most part already deepithelized. The corium remains because it is a good base for fixation sutures. The skin island can be placed in the wound to allow the perfusion to be monitored and later removed in the secondary operation for transplant correction that is usually necessary.

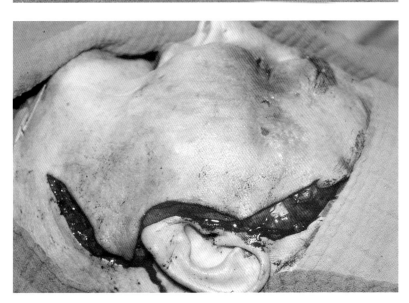

Fig. 3.**45** Preauricular S-shaped incision and undermining the skin, similar to the procedure for face lifting.

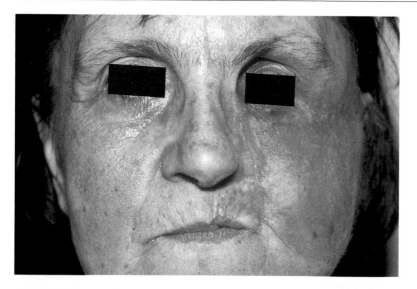

Fig. 3.**46**   Result 6 months after augmentation with the greater omentum.

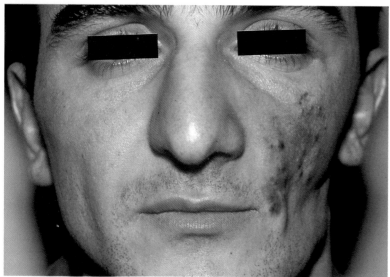

a

Fig. 3.**47**   **a** A 24-year-old patient with a subcutaneous defect of the left cheek after radiation therapy for a hemangioma in childhood. **b** Results after augmentation with a deepithelized scapular flap.

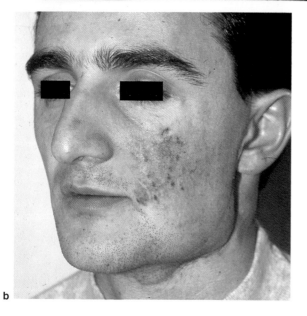

b

they provide a satisfying cosmetic result (Figs. 3.46, 3.47). As after almost all microsurgical augmentation procedures, later fine tuning of details must be carried out.

A composite bone graft (osteomyocutaneous, osteofasciocutaneous), such as the iliac crest or scapular, is well suited for bony and soft tissue defects. If bony defects accompany disorders of the positioning of the jaw or malocclusion, an osteotomy should be carried out along with the augmentation to correct the position of the jaw.

References

Anita, N., V. Buch: Transfer of an abdominal dermo-fat graft by direct anastomosis of blood vessels. Brit. J. plast. Surg. 24 (1971) 15–19

Baudet, J., J. C. Guimberteau, E. Nascimento: Successful clinical transfer of two free thoracodorsal axillary flaps. Plast. reconstr. Surg. 58 (1976) 680–688

Bootz, F., G.-H. Müller: Der radiale Unterarmlappen, seine vielseitige Anwendbarkeit in der plastischen Rekonstruktion des Kopf-Hals-Bereiches. Laryngol. Rhinol. Otol. 68 (1989) 595–601

Brown, R., F. Nahai, J. Silverton: The omentum in facial reconstruction. Brit. J. plast. Surg. 31 (1978) 58–62

Ehrenfeld, M., D. Riediger: Korrektur subkutaner Weichgewebedefekte durch mikrochirurgische Transplantate. In Schwenzer, N., G. Pfeifer: Fortschritte der Kiefer- und Gesichts-Chirurgie, Bd. XXXV: Mikrochirurgie in der Mund-, Kiefer- und Gesichts-Chirurgie. Thieme, Stuttgart 1990 (S. 100–104)

Harashima, T., T. Nakajima, Y. Yoshimura: A free groin flap reconstruction in progressive facial hemiatrophy. Brit. J. plast. Surg. 30 (1977) 14

Höltje, W. J.: Fettgewebstransplantation mit mikrochirurgischer Gefäßanastomose. In Schwenzer, N., G. Pfeifer: Fortschritte der Kiefer- und Gesichts-Chirurgie, Bd. XXXV: Mikrochirurgie in der Mund-, Kiefer- und Gesichts-Chirurgie. Thieme, Stuttgart 1990 (S. 96–100)

Mees, K., R. Baumeister, E. Kastenbauer: Mikrovaskuläre Gesichtsprofilplastik bei Hemiatrophia faciei. Laryngol. Rhinol. Otol. 67 (1988) 547–548

O'Brien, B. McC., R. Russell, W. A. Morrison, L. Sully: Burried microvascular free flap for reconstruction of soft tissue defects. Plast. reconstr. Surg. 68 (1981) 712–720

Riediger, D.: Ästhetische Gesichtspunkte bei der Versorgung von Gesichtsdefekten. In Schwenzer, N., G. Pfeifer: Fortschritte der Kiefer- und Gesichts-Chirurgie, Bd. XXXV: Ästhetische Gesichtschirurgie. Thieme, Stuttgart 1989 (S. 154–157)

Riediger, D., M. Ehrenfeld: Microsurgical Tissue Transplantation. Quintessence, Chicago 1989 (pp. 83–87)

Upten, J., J. B. Milliken, P. D. Hicks, J. E. Murray: Restoration of facial contur using free vascularized omentum. Plast. reconstr. Surg. 66 (1980) 560

Urken, M. L., H. Weinberg, C. Vickery, H. F. Biller: The neurofasciocutaneous radial forearm flap in head and neck reconstruction: a preliminary report. Laryngoscope 100 (1990) 161–173

Yang, G., B. Chen, Y. Gao, X. Liu, J. Li, S. Jiang, S. He: Forearm free skin flap transplantation. Nat. med. J. China 61 (1981) 139

4 Complications

Vascular Complications

Arterial Thrombosis

Arterial thrombosis is a feared event in microvascular surgery. It is rarer than venous thrombosis and arises either during or in the first few hours after the operation. The typical sign of arterial thrombosis is that the flap becomes white. This complication is easier to recognize in myocutaneous than in fasciocutaneous flaps. The signs of capillary filling are absent: after local pressure is applied to the flap the appearance does not change. Round objects, such as the cover of a disposable cannula pressed against the skin can be used to create a white circler as a clinical test. When the pressure is removed the capillaries fill immediately in the white circle if arterial perfusion is good, and the circle disappears within a second or less. If the arterial circulation is occluded, the white circle is barely visible and persists for several seconds. The white flap becomes patchy and gray-blue, pale in the middle, and, after a few days, necrotic.

A further test to verify arterial thrombosis is scarification: the skin is scratched with the point of a scalpel or needle. If arterial thrombosis is present, no blood appears.

Arterial thrombi are often due to poor anastomotic technique, if the vascular suture does not include all layers and the intima prolapses into the bloodstream or the opposing wall is not included in the suture. Adventitial tissue pulled into the lumen of the vessel during suturing causes a thrombus to form. The condition of the recipient and donor vessels plays an important role as well. The dissection must be carried out carefully in the receptor and donor regions: careful dissection is necessary to avoid injuries to and spasm of the vessels.

Vascular spasm is common during operation of the legs but is rare in the cervical vessels. It is usually not critical because the anastomosis is normally carried out close to the carotid artery which has sufficient blood pressure and blood flow. Physiological spasm in a traumatized vessel arises during the dissection or division as a protective mechanism in order to keep blood loss to a minimum, and is unavoidable. Normally the spasm resolves spontaneously, but if it persists after the operation it can cause ischemia of the flap.

The only sure way to brake spasm is to stretch the vessel carefully with a small Fogarty catheter. An alternative is to try to widen the aperture of the vessel with jeweler's forceps, taking care not to injure the intima. Often the situation improves just by waiting. Sometimes warmth, the external application of a local anesthetic (2% xylocain), or a calcium channel blocker can help. Local application of the calcium channel blocker verapamil is very effective.

Besides injury to vessels, local coagulation processes are also important in the genesis of thrombi. These processes are affected by the use of vessel clamps, the length of the operation, and the natural plasma and cellular coagulative processes. The pressure exerted by the clamps can damage the intima. The correct size of clamp must be used with a defined pressure adapted to the diameter of the vessel. Small changes in the vessels are "repaired" by mural thrombi that correct the endothelial damage. A change in direction of blood flow combined with local vascular damage can also result in an apposition thrombus, which can occlude the vessel. Whether perfusion of the flap with a heparin–isotonic salt solution can prevent such events is unknown but unlikely. We omit complete perfusion of the flap and rinse the arterial and venous pedicle repeatedly with a heparin solution. The solution contains 5000 units sodium heparin in 100 ml isotonic saline solution.

In addition to the apposition thrombi due to vessel wall damage and intimal separation that can result from poor suture technique, severe perfusion disorders of the flap can also be caused by twisting or kinking of the vessels. This has more significant repercussions when a vein rather than an artery is affected. If two vessels are very incongruent in size, kinks can easily occur at the anastomosis. If an anastomosis is twisted on its axis the danger of occlusion is very high. Usually the thinner vessel is twisted and causes a stenosis. This occurs at the anastomosis or at the point where the vessel is fixed to the adjacent tissue, for example where the pedicle enters the flap. If the pedicle is anastomosed when twisted more than 45°, it often cannot compensate. In such cases the anastomosis must be carried out again. Kinks can also be caused by unfavorable slanted incisions made to assist adaptation of incongruent vessels. Usually the end of the larger vessel is slanted more than that of the smaller vessel.

Kinks also occur when end-to-side anastomoses are not ideally placed. Anastomoses are particularly endangered by kinking when the flap is under pressure or tension, changing the position of the pedicle. Kinking or stretching can also be caused by severe bleeding under the flap, resulting in venous congestion and then arterial compromise which endangers the flap.

The management of arterial thrombosis consists of exposure and revision of the anastomosis. Two or three sutures are removed from the anastomosis to allow inspection of the vessel lumen. In some cases the thrombus can be removed. Sutures that are technically inadequate should be removed and renewed. The ends of the vessels must be shortened to produce a smooth cut edge for the reanastomosis. The procedure for removing an apposition thrombus in the recipient vessel is complicated. The vessel is irrigated under minimal pressure with the anastomosis fully open. Alternatively the thrombus can be bypassed by a small Fogarty catheter to try to pull the thrombus out of the vessel with the balloon, but there is a danger of pushing the thrombus further into the vessel. Size 2 Fogarty catheters are used in free tissue transplantation. The careful use of this catheter combined with intensive irrigation in a heparin–isotonic saline solution can be successful.

If the cause of the occlusion cannot be found, heparin should be administered systemically after using the Fogarty catheter. In our experience this is necessary for mural thrombi. In order to prevent the intravascular pressure from rising too high during irrigation, we always irrigate the artery when it is open. Most of the solution can

then flow out of the inflow region and the opening of the anastomosis. After successful revision we administer heparin systemically using a perfusion device. Between 25000 and 35000 units per day are necessary to achieve a PTT of 50 seconds.

The damage that can result from ischemia is different for the different cell systems and depends on time. Interruption of the circulation to skin, muscle, or bone for up to 8 hours does not cause any functional damage. This time interval must be kept in mind during postoperative monitoring, since revision of vascular anastomosis during this time after vascular complications is most likely to be successful.

Venous Thrombosis

The classic picture of a venous thrombosis is the blue flap (Fig. 4.1a). The phase of venous thrombosis is marked by an increase in number of petechiae on the surface of the skin. The longer the occlusion is present the more they increase, particularly at the edges of the transplant. The flap first becomes red, then purple, and finally blue. Once the flap swells the situation becomes critical. The color of the vessel wall during the operation indicates whether the anastomosis is insufficient or the outflow is deficient from the recipient vessel. Darkening or ballooning of the flap vein is always the first sign of an outflow disorder.

Venous thrombi are caused either by an unsatisfactory anastomotic technique or by postoperative complications. The most common technical errors are twisting and kinking of the pedicles in relation to each other. Additional damage to the wall of the vein due to inadequate suture technique, or injury by vascular clamps or microinstruments can also be causes of thrombi. A high risk of venous thrombosis is always present when adventitial tissue such as fat gets into the vessel lumen due to poor anastomotic technique. Apposition thrombi are common and can completely occlude a vein. Postoperative development of kinks in the vein at the anastomosis is particularly a hazard in end-to-side anastomosis. High tension on a vessel can cause occlusion when even a very small change in position occurs.

Another cause of venous thrombosis is postoperative bleeding (p. 89) from the anastomosis itself, or more often from the edges of the transplant, such as from the divided muscle in a myocutaneous flap.

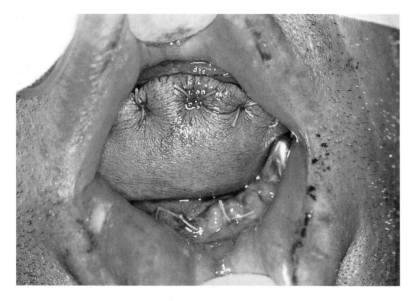

Fig. 4.**1 a–c**   Venous stasis in a fore-arm flap. **a** A blue flap about 4 hours after the operation.

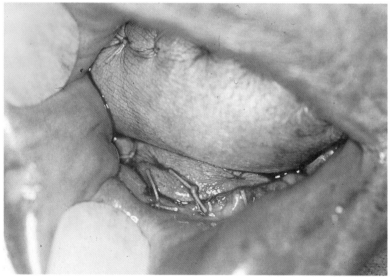

b   Immediately after the revision a significant improvement in the venous flow is already apparent.

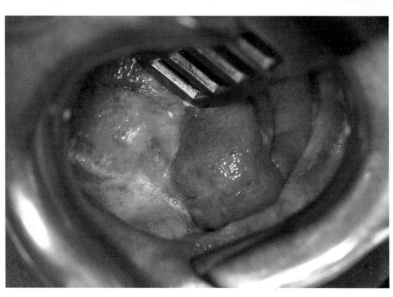

c   Appearance 6 months after the operation and radiation therapy.

If venous thrombosis has occurred the vessels must be exposed and the anastomosis opened to eliminate the cause. The vein must be carefully catheterized and rinsed with a heparin–isotonic saline solution. After removing two or three sutures the artery is irrigated until the solution appears in the venous limb of the pedicle. It is often possible to improve the flap's perfusion by this technique (Figs. **4.1b,c**). In these cases we carry out postoperative heparinization. If the obstruction was due to bleeding complete hemostasis is achieved after the hematoma has been evacuated and the wound drained. After every revision the usual perfusion tests are done on the vessel. The Acland test has proven to be the most useful for judging venous patency (p. 58). We do not use special flowmeters or microdoppler devices.

References

Black, M. J. M., L. Chait, B. McC. O'Brien, P. J. Sykes, L. A. Sharzer: How soon may the axial vessels of a surviving free flap be safely ligated? A study in pigs. Brit. J. plast. Surg. 31 (1978) 295

Khoo, C. T. K., B. N. Bailey: The behaviour of free muscle and musculocutaneous flaps after early loss of axial blood supply. Brit. J. plast. Surg. 35 (1982) 43–46

Nakajima, T.: How soon do venous drainage channels develop at the periphery of a free flap? A study in rats. Brit. J. plast. Surg. 31 (1978) 300

Serafin, D., J. C. Shearin, N. G. Georgiade: The vascularization of free flaps. Plast. reconstr. Surg. 60 (1977) 233

Smith, P. J.: The importance of venous drainage in axial pattern flaps. Brit. J. plast. Surg. 31 (1978) 233

Bleeding

Bleeding can complicate every vascular procedure. Bleeding can stem from the anastomosis, the pedicle, the transplanted tissue itself, or the transplant bed. The musculocutaneous flaps must be mentioned (Fig. **4.2**) in particular, because of the brisk bleeding from the edges of the transplanted muscle. However, the edges of fasciocutaneous flaps often bleed also, particularly

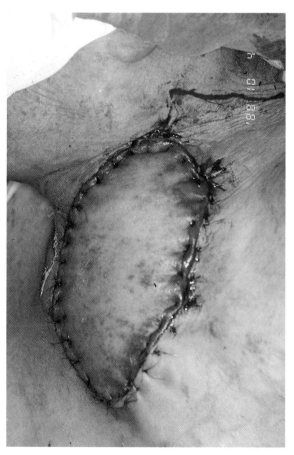

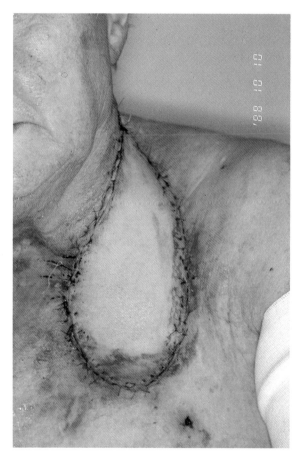

Fig. **4.2 a** Combined disturbed arterial and venous circulation in a latissimus dorsi flap, caused by bleeding in the graft bed.

b Normal perfusion 6 days after revision and hemostasis.

when they have been harvested, as frequently recommended, with the use of a tourniquet. We omit the tourniquet for this reason.

In some cases bleeding can occur simply because the flap has changed its position, exerting tension on the pedicle that leads to occlusion. The increasing narrowing of the vein correlates with an increased volume of the flap, leading to a vicious circle, which compromises the arterial perfusion, and encourages the development of thrombi. An immediate revision is absolutely necessary in such cases.

Bleeding must be taken seriously because it can lead to kinking of vessels and the development of thrombi. It is important to ensure sufficient drainage from the undersurface of the flap from the very beginning of the procedure. Meticulous hemostasis during flap elevation and intraoperative control of bleeding during anastomosis of vessels reduce the risk of bleeding. After some unfortunate experiences we have stopped administering anticoagulants as a routine and we do not even use platelet aggregation inhibitors such as aspirin. Occasionally dextran can be used to improve the perfusion of the capillary beds. After the first day 500 ml dextran 40 is administered as an infusion for 4 hours daily for 5 days. Low-dose heparin is given to immobilized patients.

Bleeding from the bone edges also is dangerous when the drainage is inadequate; bone wax is useful in these cases. The Jackson–Pratt and usual suction drains are helpful. Passive drains, such as the Penrose and Easy-flow drains, can be used for fasciocutaneous flaps. The drain must not be placed next to the anastomosis. It is important when removing the drains to release the active suction by allowing air to enter the drain.

Although bleeding from muscle and bone can usually be controlled with drains, postoperative bleeding as seen in intestinal transplants is more difficult. This is true for bleeding from the mesentery as well as the intestinal mucosa.

In the latter case it is usually better to wait and coagulation factors might need correction. If the bleeding is not stemmed by these methods, the anastomosis should be reexposed and if necessary, redone, in order to protect the transplant.

Bleeding is particularly dangerous for intestinal loops from which the mucosa has been removed. If it is not arrested, secondary bleeding can endanger the graft. It can be just as difficult to control bleeding from a deepithelized skin flap. Control of the edges of the wound after anastomosis of the vessels with hemostasis should secure the situation. In some cases the vessels must be anastomized before the final positioning and implantation of the flap is carried out.

Complications at the Donor Site

The question as to whether the donor site can be closed in a functionally and aesthetically satisfying manner plays a large part in the choice of tissue to be transplanted. Microvascular tissue transplantation is the best and surest way to rehabilitate the patient quickly but it should not be done at the cost of a significant donor defect. A donor defect that can be closed primarily is to be distinguished from one that must be covered with a split skin graft. The scar is always visible after primary closure if it is done under tension: the greater the tension the broader the scar. A primary closure is not always possible with fasciocutaneous flaps.

The simplest and functionally most satisfactory cover for the defect after harvesting a dorsalis pedis or a forearm flap can be achieved with a thick split skin graft. Split skin is not comparable to original skin because of its more intensive pigmentation and its limited ability to withstand stress. Donor defects after the use of forearm and dorsalis pedis flaps are difficult particularly when the split skin does not heal primarily. If tendons are exposed while elevating the flap, the paratenon must be protected. In order to prevent the split skin from shearing over the tendon we recommend immobilization using a volar plaster splint for the forearm flap and a plaster splint on the lower leg for the dorsalis pedis flap. If the split skin becomes necrotic, particularly over the tendon of the flexor carpi radialis muscle (Fig. 4.3 a), we wait for the granulation process to begin spontaneously; if the region is inflammation-free a new split skin graft can be applied (Fig. 4.3 b,c).

If a tendon undergoes necrosis, necrotic tissue must be excised from the dry area of the tendon before a new transplant can be used for coverage. Seromas and hematomas lead to infection and abnormal wound healing, particularly between the projecting tendons of the first and second metatarsals, after removal of a dorsalis pedis flap. If possible, a mesh graft should not be used to cover the defect, but rather a thick split skin graft elevated in one piece. To facilitate this we make a template of the defect on the forearm

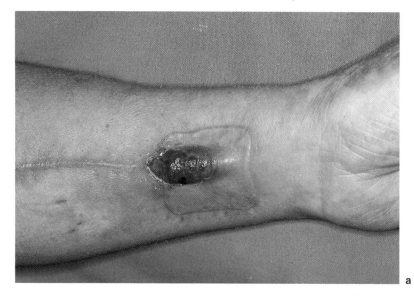

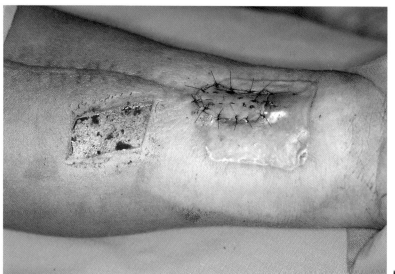

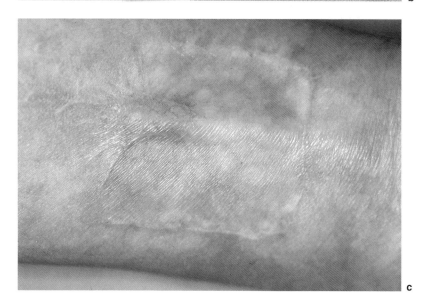

Fig. 4.**3 a**   Defect over the tendon
of the flexor carpi radialis muscle
with granulation tissue formation.
b Application of a new split skin graft.
c Satisfactory result 3 months later.

or the foot and cut the split skin to size from an over-large piece cut with a dermatome. Exact defect coverage can usually be achieved. Skin clips that are usually used for split skin grafts are not suitable for this reconstruction, and we use interrupted sutures instead. Over the dorsum of the foot a bolus dressing can be helpful. It is removed after 5 days to ensure that no infection is overlooked. By this time the split skin should have healed to its bed.

In order to improve the cosmetic results of the donor defect on the forearm attempts have been made to use an ulnar fasciocutaneous advancement flap for closure. However, since this demands yet another invasion of the soft tissue of the forearm, it should only be carried out with small forearm flaps.

Secondary complications after fasciocutaneous flaps include superficial sensory disturbances. This is to be expected due to division of the cutaneous antibrachii nerve or the superficial branch of the radial nerve in the forearm flap or in the area of the dorsalis pedis flap after lesions of the dorsal cutaneous nerves.

We have never seen vascular complications at the donor site affecting the foot or forearm. We do not consider vessel reconstruction by a vein graft to be indicated. The patency of such grafts after reconstructing the radial artery is about 50%. Careful preoperative assessment identifies patients in whom postoperative perfusion disorders can be expected (p. 56).

Early complications after the elevation of myocutaneous flaps include bleeding and infection. Although bleeding from the vessel stumps is rare, it is not uncommon from the muscle remaining after a partial resection to form a muscle flap. This is not only due to inadequate technique: after tissue removal, the small vessels that are opened do not bleed at first but after some time bleed intensely due to the increased quantity of blood draining distal to this region. Therefore we suture the remaining edges of the muscle.

Functional impairment can follow removal of the rectus abdominis flap. Because the rectus muscle is needed for breathing, the lung function is impaired, particularly in older patients. There is also the danger of hernia development. We use reabsorbable net (Dexon) to reinforce the lower part of what was once the rectus sheath to prevent hernia formation.

Hypertrophic scars are another complication arising at the donor site of the rectus abdominis muscle. If the edges of the wound have to be su-tured under tension, dehiscence and infection are more common. Although they can be treated conservatively, the cooperation of the patient is necessary, and hospitalization must be extended. Wound dehiscence in the area of the rectus muscle, particularly at the edges of the fascia, can lead to the development of a hernia. If dehiscence is limited to the cutis, secondary healing can be expected.

Elevation of the latissimus dorsi muscle usually causes no significant functional impairment but the defect leaves a visible scar, particularly when a split skin graft is used for closure (Fig. 4.4). The scars are rarely aesthetically satisfactory because they usually broaden, and women especially should be warned of this before the operation.

We always treat wound dehiscence at the donor site for the latissimus dorsi muscle conservatively (Fig. 4.5). We use a mesh graft to cover the defect after stabilizing the edges of the wound and cleaning the wound bed. Such defects usually heal in 2 to 3 weeks.

The correct use of drains can help avoid complications. After elevating a latissimus dorsi flap, two suction drains are placed parallel to each other. We use the same principle after lifting a rectus abdominis flap, but place one drain between the anterior and posterior rectus sheath, even when it is dry.

Elevation of an osteomyocutaneous flap can cause instability in the bony structure, be it of the iliac crest, scapula, or first metatarsal. We have reported a fracture after elevation of an osteofasciocutaneous forearm flap. An instability in the middle foot after removal of the second metatarsal bone in a dorsalis pedis flap is also possible. Fractures are unlikely in the area of the iliac crest or scapula. We have seen a rare complication 2 years after elevation of an iliac crest graft: an aneurysm developed in the external iliac artery and had to be surgically removed.

Infection is a serious complication after elevation of osteomyocutaneous flaps. The principles of septic trauma surgery must be followed, using closed irrigation–suction drains after excision of necrotic tissue, sequestrectomy, immobilization, and antibiotic therapy. After elevation of a bowel loop or the omentum, a burst abdomen can lead to complications. This is common after infection, which is frequent after intestinal surgery. We have never encountered problems with anastomosis of the small intestine, but they are possible. Early infections in the abdominal wound should be treated locally, and inflamed

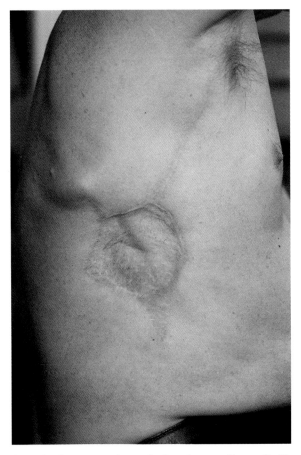

Fig. 4.4   Poor cosmetic result after closure with a split skin graft of a donor defect arising from the use of a latissimus dorsi flap.

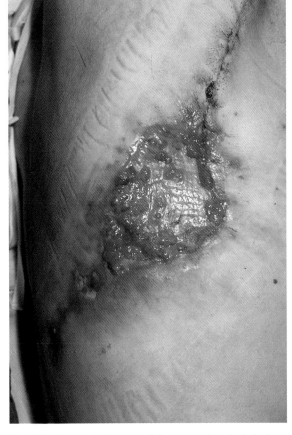

Fig. 4.5   Suture dehiscence at the donor site of a latissimus dorsi flap with secondary wound healing and formation of granulation tissue.

wounds must be regularly inspected. If there is a suspicion of infection, the wound must be opened and drained.

The spread of infection must be prevented as this can lead to a secondary hernia.

Complications in the anastomosis of the intestine depend on the technique chosen. We prefer a single-layer suture, which scarcely affects the perfusion of the small intestine and ensures secure closure even of wide anastomoses. An intestinal stenosis can be a further complication. A secondary mechanical ileus is rare after a single-layer intestinal suture, but a secondary ileus due to adhesions is more common. We do not recommend drains after anastomosis of the small intestine. Sometimes an indicator probe is inserted on the first day after the operation as a drain for bleeding.

We have rarely seen complications after harvesting the omentum. If the procedure was technically correct it can be assumed that the transverse colon or stomach have not been injured.

Sometimes smaller sources of bleeding give rise to an intra-abdominal hematoma, particularly around the omentum after partial resection. Bleeding from the spleen is a serious complication that can arise in any operation in the upper abdomen. Dissection of the arcade of vessels along the greater curvature of the stomach must be meticulous, otherwise postoperative bleeding from this area can be considerable. We do not use any special postoperative care. Intestinal function should be back to normal within 2 days of removal of the omentum.

Free tissue transfers always leave a permanent defect at the donor site. The extent of the defect should always be in proportion to the value of the reconstruction. If functional considerations are more important than appearance, a cosmetic defect at the donor site can be acceptable. Patients who have undergone reconstructive surgery after resection of a tumor of the upper aerodigestive tract repeatedly endorse our opinion: restoration of function is their greatest priority.

References

Boorman, J. G., J. A. Brown, P. J. Sykes: Morbidity in the forearm flap donor arm. Brit. J. plast. Surg. 40 (1987) 207–212

Bootz, F., E. Biesinger: Reduction of complication rate at radial forearm flap donor site. Oto-Rhino-Laryngol. 53 (1990) 160–164

Fenton, O. M., J. O. Roberts: Improving the donor site of the radial forearm flap. Brit. J. plast. Surg. 38 (1985) 504–505

Jones, B. M., C. J. O'Brien: Acute ischaemia of the hand resulting from elevation of a radial forearm flap. Brit. J. plast. Surg. 38 (1985) 396–397

McGregor, A. D.: The free radial forearm flap – the management of the secondary defect. Brit. J. plast. Surg. 40 (1987) 83–85

Swanson, C., J. B. Boyd, R. T. Manktelow: The radial forearm flap: reconstructive applications and donor-site defects in 35 consecutive patients. Plast. reconstr. Surg. 85 (1990) 258–266

Timmons, M. J., F. E. M. Missotten, M. D. Poole, D. M. Davies: Complications of radial forearm flap donor sites. Brit. J. plast. Surg. 39 (1986) 176–178

Further References

Textbooks

Acland, R. D.: Microsurgery, Practice Manual. Mosby, St. Louis 1980

Berger, A., C. Tizian: Technik der Mikrochirurgie. Lehrbuch und Atlas. Kohlhammer, Stuttgart 1985

Biemer, E., W. Duspiva: Rekonstruktive Mikrogefäßchirurgie. Springer, Berlin 1980

Conley, J., C. Patow: Flaps in Head and Neck Surgery, 2nd ed. Thieme, Stuttgart 1989

Cormack, G. C., B. G. H. Lamberty: The Arterial Anatomy of Skin Flaps. Churchill Livingstone, Edinburgh 1986

Harii, K.: Microvascular Tissue Transfer. Fundamental Techniques and Clinical Applications. Igaku-Shoin, Tokyo 1983

Manktelow, R. T.: Mikrovaskuläre Wiederherstellungschirurgie. Springer, Berlin 1988

McCraw, J. B., P. G. Arnold: McCraw and Arnold's Atlas of Muscle and Musculocutaneous Flaps. Hampton Press, Norfolk,Va. 1986

Mehdorn, H. M., G. H. Müller: Mikrochirurgische Übungen. Thieme, Stuttgart 1987

O'Brien, B. McC., W. A. Morrison: Reconstructive Microsurgery. Churchill Livingstone, Edinburgh 1987

Panje, W. R., W. J. Moran: Free Flap Reconstruction of the Head and Neck. Thieme, Stuttgart 1989

Riediger, D.: Mikrochirurgische Weichgewebetransplantation in die Gesichtsregion. Experiment und Klinik. Hanser, München 1983

Serafin, D., H. J. Buncke jr.: Microsurgical Composite Tissue Transplantation. Mosby, St. Louis 1979

Strauch, B., H.-L. Yu: Atlas of Microvascular Surgery. Anatomy and Operative Approaches. Thieme Medical Publishers, New York 1993

Webster, M., D. Soutar: Practical Guide to Free Tissue Transfer. Butterworth, London 1986

Journals

British Journal of Plastic Surgery. Livingstone, Edinburgh

Handchirurgie, Mikrochirurgie, Plastische Chirurgie. Hippokrates, Stuttgart

Plastic and Reconstructive Surgery. Williams & Wilkins, Baltimore

Reconstructive Microsurgery. Thieme, New York

Index

Page numbers in *italics* refer to figures